# Adult T-cell Leukemia/Lymphoma

Toshiki Watanabe • Takuya Fukushima
Editors

# Adult T-cell Leukemia/Lymphoma

Springer

*Editors*
Toshiki Watanabe
Department of Medical Genome Sciences
Graduate School of Frontier Sciences
The University of Tokyo
Tokyo, Japan

Takuya Fukushima
Department of Clinical Laboratory Sciences
School of Health Sciences
University of the Ryukyus
Okinawa, Japan

ISBN 978-4-431-56521-5 ISBN 978-4-431-56523-9 (eBook)
DOI 10.1007/978-4-431-56523-9

Library of Congress Control Number: 2017936208



Printed on acid-free paper

This Springer imprint is published by Springer Nature
The registered company is Springer Japan KK
The registered company address is: Chiyoda First Bldg. East, 3-8-1 Nishi-Kanda, Chiyoda-ku, Tokyo 101-0065, Japan

# Standardization of Terminology

## Formal Name of HTLV-1

The formal name of HTLV-1 is "human T-cell leukaemia virus type I" or "human T-lymphotropic virus type I". In principle, the name of an animal retrovirus should be specified using the name of the disease initially associated with the virus. Furthermore, we regard "lymphotropic" as an improper name for HTLV-1 because the HTLV-1 receptor on the cell surface is not cell-type specific, and it has been shown that HTLV-1 infects not only lymphocytes but also several other kinds of cells. For these reasons, we have adopted "human T-cell leukaemia virus type I" as the formal name for HTLV-1 in this book.

## Abbreviation of Adult T-Cell Leukaemia-Lymphoma

In the first report on adult T-cell leukaemia-lymphoma, Uchiyama et al. focused on 16 patients with leukaemic cells in peripheral blood and called the disease "adult T-cell leukaemia". Therefore, "ATL" was initially used as the abbreviation for the disease. It was subsequently revealed that some patients had lymphoma-type disease, which led to the general understanding that this disease is a subtype of peripheral T-cell lymphoma. Thus, "adult T-cell leukaemia-lymphoma" became the common disease name, and "ATLL" has also been used as an abbreviation. The WHO Classification of Tumours of Haematopoietic and Lymphoid Tissues (2008) uses "ATLL", but both "ATL" and "ATLL" are now generally accepted. In this book, we adopt the initial name of this disease, and these abbreviations of adult T-cell leukaemia-lymphoma are consolidated to "ATL".

# Contents

1 **Overview** . . . . . . . . . . 1
Toshiki Watanabe and Takuya Fukushima

2 **Human T-Cell Leukemia Virus Type 1 (HTLV-1)** . . . . . . . . . . 3
Jun-ichi Fujisawa

3 **Epidemiology** . . . . . . . . . . 33
Masako Iwanaga

4 **Pathology** . . . . . . . . . . 49
Koichi Ohshima and Hiroaki Miyoshi

5 **Immunophenotype** . . . . . . . . . . 67
Kaoru Uchimaru

6 **Leukemogenesis and Molecular Characteristics of Tumor Cells** . . . . . . . . . . 83
Toshiki Watanabe

7 **Clinical Features of Adult T-cell Leukemia/Lymphoma (ATL)** . . . 101
Yoshitaka Imaizumi

8 **Prognosis and Prognostic Index** . . . . . . . . . . 109
Takuya Fukushima

9 **Treatment of Indolent Adult T-cell Leukemia/Lymphoma (ATL)** . . . . . . . . . . 117
Kenji Ishitsuka

10 **Chemotherapy of Aggressive Adult T-cell Leukemia/Lymphoma (ATL)** . . . . . . . . . . 125
Kunihiro Tsukasaki

**11 Transplantation for Aggressive Adult T-Cell Leukemia/Lymphoma (ATL)** . . . . . . . . . . . . . . . . . . . . . . . . . . . . . 133
Atae Utsunomiya

**12 New Agents of Adult T-cell Leukemia/Lymphoma (ATL)** . . . . . . . . 145
Wataru Munakata and Kensei Tobinai

**13 Prevention of Human T-Cell Leukemia Virus Type 1 (HTLV-1) Mother-to-Child Transmission** . . . . . . . . . . . . . . 157
Kiyonori Miura and Hideaki Masuzaki

# Chapter 1
# Overview

**Toshiki Watanabe and Takuya Fukushima**

The disease entity of adult T-cell leukemia-lymphoma (ATL) was proposed by Takatsuki et al. in 1977, and human T-cell leukemia virus type I (HTLV-1) was discovered as the causative virus of ATL in the early 1980s. Since then, many researchers—especially in Japan where it is endemic with the highest prevalence in the world—have been investigating and clarifying its many features including the epidemiology of HTLV-1, the molecular mechanisms of the progression from HTLV-1 infection to ATL, and the development of more effective treatment for ATL.

In the field of basic research, the start was the clarification of the whole structure of HTLV-1 genes. A large amount of evidence has accumulated about the function of viral gene products such as Tax, Rex, antisense RNA/protein HBZ, and others, which has led to a new concept of pathogenetic roles for development of ATL and other associated diseases. Characterization of HTLV-1-infected cells and their clonal growth in vivo has provided a new insight into the behavior of HTLV-1-infected T cells. ATL develops based on the multistep carcinogenesis model involving five or more genetic events. Recent studies using new technologies such as next-generation sequencing have provided a series of new results about genetic and epigenetic abnormalities underlying ATL leukemogenesis including those underlying the progression from HTLV-1 carrier status to ATL and from indolent ATL to aggressive ATL. The results also provided possible targets for molecularly targeted therapies.

T. Watanabe (✉)
Department of Medical Genome Sciences, Graduate School of Frontier Sciences, The University of Tokyo, Tokyo, Japan
e-mail: tnabe@marianna-u.ac.jp

T. Fukushima
Department of Clinical Laboratory Sciences, School of Health Sciences, University of the Ryukyus, Okinawa, Japan
e-mail: fukutaku@med.u-ryukyu.ac.jp



T. Watanabe, T. Fukushima (eds.), *Adult T-cell Leukemia/Lymphoma*,
DOI 10.1007/978-4-431-56523-9_1

In the clinical field, clinical trials of therapy for aggressive ATL have been conducted after the establishment of the clinical classification by Shimoyama et al., and a 5-year overall survival of aggressive ATL has improved from 5% in the 1980s to 15% in the 1990s. Mogamulizumab, a defucosylated anti-CC chemokine receptor 4 antibody, was approved for relapsed ATL from 2012 and untreated ATL from 2014 by the Ministry of Health, Labour and Welfare in Japan, and combination therapy with antineoplastic agents is expected to improve the survival outcome of patients with aggressive ATL. Moreover, allogeneic hematopoietic stem cell transplantation, which has been applied to aggressive ATL actively from the 1990s, has demonstrated a better outcome than standard chemotherapy and provided the possibility of cure in some patients with aggressive ATL.

To establish a comprehensive strategy against HTLV-1 infection and HTLV-1-associated diseases, HTLV-1 comprehensive methods were started from 2010 in Japan. Moreover, the Japanese Society of HTLV-1 was founded in 2013 followed by the Japanese Workshop of HTLV-1, and research combining and utilizing both basic science and clinical medicine is accelerating.

This book about HTLV-1 and ATL was written by experts of epidemiology, basic science, and clinical medicine and includes recent knowledge about the disease. We truly appreciate all authors and also the efforts of the staff in Springer Japan. We believe that this book will provide many insights for clinicians and basic researchers.

# Chapter 2
# Human T-Cell Leukemia Virus Type 1 (HTLV-1)

**Jun-ichi Fujisawa**

## 2.1 Human T-Cell Leukemia Virus Type 1 (HTLV-1) as the First Human Retrovirus

Within several decades after identification of the first retroviruses as agents of neoplastic diseases in chickens at the beginning of last century [36, 150], a large number of "RNA tumor virus" were found in fowl, mice, cat, cattle, and monkeys. In addition to the extraordinary and unique features of life cycle such as reverse transcription of genomic RNA to DNA and its integration into the host chromosomal DNA, analysis of retroviruses led to the finding of "oncogenes" and provided a strong evidence for the paradigm, the genetic origin of cancer. However, retroviruses had been searched for without success in most types of human tumors by the end of the 1970s; thus, it seemed questionable whether a human retrovirus existed at all.

In 1980, the first human retrovirus was found in a T-cell line established from a patient with mycosis fungoides, and the retrovirus was named human T-cell leukemia virus type I (HTLV-1) [145], but the link between this retrovirus and human disease was not certain. Prior to this finding, Takatsuki and his colleague reported a new disease entity, adult T-cell leukemia (ATL). Patients with ATL were clustered in a limited area of Japan, including the islands of Kyushu and Okinawa, which suggested a transmissible leukemogenic agent [178]. A large number of T-cell lines, so-called ATL cell lines, were established from ATL patients, and it was found that all ATL patients had antibodies that reacted with these cell lines, confirming the involvement of virus infection [65]. Subsequently, a retrovirus particle was identified in the ATL cell line [127], and the nucleotide sequence of the retrovirus, initially called ATLV, was determined [154, 193]. Comparison of

J.-i. Fujisawa (✉)
Department of Microbiology, Kansai Medical University, 2-5-1 Shin-machi, Hirakata, Osaka 573-1010, Japan
e-mail: fujisawa@hirakata.kmu.ac.jp



T. Watanabe, T. Fukushima (eds.), *Adult T-cell Leukemia/Lymphoma*,
DOI 10.1007/978-4-431-56523-9_2

the nucleotide sequences between HTLV-1 and ATLV revealed that these two viruses were almost identical [186].

Cloning of the HTLV-1 genome provided a molecular tool to prove the close association of HTLV-1 infection to ATL. First, the HTLV-1 provirus was detected without exception in the genome of leukemic cells from ATL patients. Second, a majority of leukemic cell from a given patient harbored the provirus at the same chromosomal site in the genome, indicating monoclonal growth of the infected cell; otherwise, the integration would occur at random in the natural retrovirus infection. Thus, it was concluded that HTLV-1 is a causative agent of ATL [154].

Nucleotide sequencing of its viral genome showed that HTLV-1 lacked a cell-derived oncogene, yet it was more complex than other oncogenic retroviruses [154]. Integration sites of the provirus in leukemic cells from different ATL patients, however, differ from each other, demonstrating the absence of insertional activation of a cellular oncogene. The two well-known mechanisms of retroviral oncogenesis, transduction and cis-activation of an oncogene, therefore did not apply to HTLV-1.

In addition to essential structural and enzymatic genes (*gag*, *pro*, *pol*, and *env*) shared by all retroviral family members [92], HTLV-1 encodes a unique pX region, which generates two regulatory (Tax, Rex) and five accessory (HBZ, p30, p12, p13, p8) proteins [25, 100]. Among them, Tax and HBZ have been shown to play pivotal roles in the viral life cycle and affect expression levels of several host genes [38, 125, 159]. Therefore, a new type of oncogenic mechanism by retrovirus, in which viral transforming proteins other than viral or cellular oncogene are involved, was presented in the development of ATL.

## 2.2 Genome Structure and Replication of HTLV-1

### *2.2.1 Structural Genes*

A full-length mRNA, which is identical to genomic RNA, is translated mainly to produce a Gag precursor protein (PrGag, p55). After being assembled with genomic RNA to form viral particle, PrGag is processed by viral protease (PR) to produce the matrix (MA; p19), the capsid (CA; p24), and the nucleocapsid (NC; p15) proteins (Fig. 2.1b).

The *pro* and *pol* gene products were produced by the proteolytic cleavage of Gag-Pro and Gag-Pro-Pol fusion proteins translated from the same full-length mRNA by one and two successive slip-back of reading frame (frameshifts), respectively. Viral protease further separates the Pol protein (p98) into the reverse transcriptase (RT; p62) and integrase enzymes (IN; p49) (Fig. 2.1a).

The *env* message is a singly spliced mRNA, removing the gag and pol genes as an intron from the mRNA. The *env* mRNA is translated to a precursor Env protein and the protein is glycosylated and trimerized in the endoplasmic reticulum (ER).

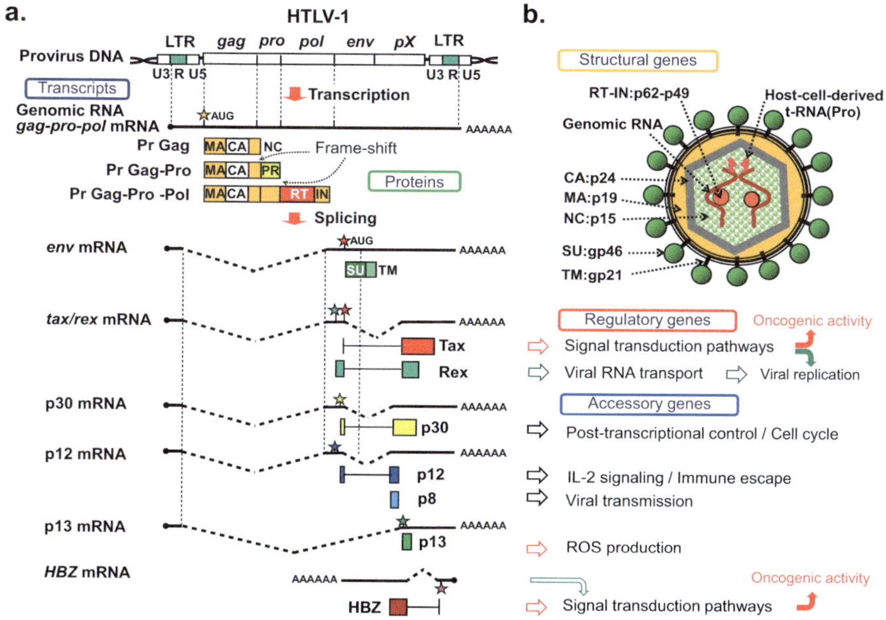


**Fig. 2.1** HTLV-1 genome structure and expression of viral genes. (**a**) Schematic organization of HTLV-1 proviral DNA (*upper*), its transcripts (*lower*), and their translated products (*lower right*) are presented. (**b**) Structure of HTLV-1 virion and function of regulatory and accessory gene products

The precursor, gp68, is then cleaved by cellular protease, furin, to form the separate surface (SU; gp46) and transmembrane (TM; p21) subunits [61] (Fig. 2.1b). Cell receptor-binding activity is conferred by gp46 and the fusion activity is a function of gp21.

### 2.2.2 *Regulatory Proteins: Tax and Rex*

Tax and Rex are essential for efficient HTLV-1 replication and production, since HTLV-1 mutants lacking either Tax or Rex function are not able to replicate in vitro as well as in vivo [148].

Both Tax and Rex proteins are translated from an identical doubly spliced *tax/rex* mRNA species using different initiation codons and reading frames of translation. Tax is a transcriptional activator of HTLV-1 and thus further amplifies the HTLV-1 transcripts, mostly spliced forms, by augmenting transcriptional activity of the long terminal repeat (LTR). Once the other product, Rex, accumulates in a sufficient amount, it enhances the export of singly spliced *env* mRNA and unspliced genomic RNA encoding *gag/pro-pol*, leading to the formation of HTLV-1 particle. Nuclear export of primary unspliced and singly spliced transcripts, in turn, results in

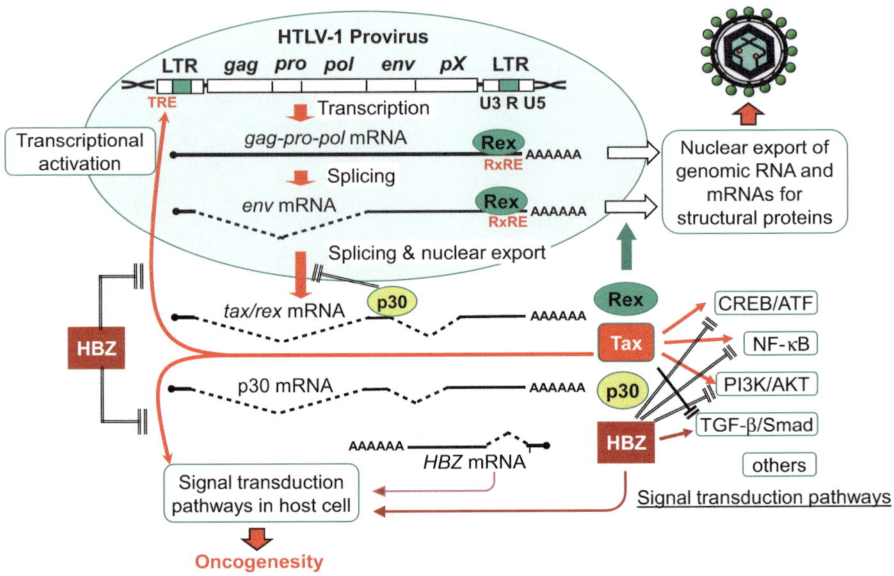


**Fig. 2.2** Control of viral and cellular gene expression by viral gene products. Upon initial infection, doubly spliced mRNAs for *tax/rex* gene are dominantly expressed. Tax first augments viral transcription by indirect binding to TRE sequence in the HTLV-1 long terminal repeat (*LTR*) promoter, and this activity is negatively regulated by HBZ. Rex enhances the nuclear export of unspliced and singly spliced mRNAs though binding to the RxRE sequence at the 3′ end of unspliced and singly spliced mRNA, thereby increasing the translation of structural proteins, resulting in HTLV-1 virion production. p30 binds to the splice junction of *tax/rex* mRNA and inhibits its nuclear export. In addition, Tax and HBZ modulate a variety of cellular signaling pathways, leading to accelerated cell proliferation and induction of genome lesions. In most pathways, HBZ has opposite effects to Tax

the reduction of doubly spliced *tax/rex* mRNA, thereby causing the temporal cessation of transcriptional activation (Fig. 2.2).

In addition to activation of viral transcription, Tax plays pivotal roles in HTLV-1 immortalization of T cells, persistent infection, inflammation, and pathogenesis, as discussed in the following sections. Rex is essential for persistent HTLV-1 infection in rabbits but not required for immortalization of human T cells in vitro [191].

#### 2.2.2.1 Transcriptional Activation of LTR by Tax

Tax protein of 353 amino acids long activates HTLV-1 transcription through LTR. Three highly conserved 21-bp repeat elements located within the U3 region of the LTR are critical to Tax-mediated transcriptional activation, thus referred to as Tax-responsive element (TRE) [22, 37, 42]. The TRE contains an octamer motif TGACG(T/A)(C/G)(T/A) that shares homology with the consensus cAMP-responsive element (CRE) 5′-TGACGTCA-3′ [43, 75], and a number of proteins of the CRE-binding/activating family of transcription factors (CREB/ATF) bind to this sequence [175, 194]. Tax does not bind directly to the TRE element [44, 48] but interacts with members of CREB/ATF family, including CREB, CREM, ATF1, ATF2, ATF3, ATF4 (CREB2), and XBP1 (X-box-binding protein 1) [10, 40, 103, 112, 146, 162, 197].

Among them, CREB plays a major role in the transcriptional activation of LTR. CREB regulates several cellular genes, especially cAMP-responsive genes, and cAMP signal leads to the phosphorylation of CREB at serine 133, recruiting coactivators (CBP/p300 and P/CAF) to facilitate transcriptional initiation. The direct interaction of Tax with CBP allows the binding of the coactivator in the absence of CREB phosphorylation [104]; however, strong Tax binding to CPB/p300 requires TRE DNA and phosphorylated CREB [94]. On the other hand, Tax expression directly enhances CREB phosphorylation in vivo to ensure availability for Tax transactivation [94].

Tax also binds to CREB coactivator proteins called transducers of regulated CREB activity (TORC1, TORC2, and TORC3) [27, 72] and TORCs cooperate with Tax to activate the LTR in a CREB and p300-dependent manner [97, 158]. Downregulation of TORC2 through its phosphorylation is associated with the in vivo specific transcriptional repression of HTLV-1 LTR [78].

#### 2.2.2.2 Posttranscriptional Regulation of Viral RNA by Rex

In addition to genomic unspliced mRNA encoding *gag/pol*, HTLV-1 expresses multiple mRNAs with distinctive splicings [155]. Three different singly spliced mRNAs encode *env*, *p12* and *p13*, respectively, and two doubly spliced mRNAs are for *tax/rex* and *p30* (Fig. 2.1).

Upon initial infection of host cells, primary transcripts with introns generally undergo splicing by the cellular RNA machinery, resulting in the preferential expression of doubly spliced *tax/rex* and *p30* mRNAs. Once the Rex protein accumulates, Rex binds specifically to the HTLV-1 RNA at the Rex-responsive element (RxRE) located in the U3 and R regions of the 3′ LTR [17, 179], through the interaction with a long stem-loop structure in the RxRE [18, 174]. Then Rex interacts with the nuclear export receptor protein CRM1/exportin 1, which mediates the transport of viral mRNAs from the nucleus to the cytoplasm, by the function of a typical leucine-rich nuclear export signal (NES) in Rex (aa81–94) [54]. Thus, Rex increases the amount of singly spliced (*env*) and unspliced (*gag-pol*) mRNAs and reduces the amount of its own doubly spliced mRNA by inhibiting the splicing of simply spliced (*env*, *p12*, *p13*, and *p21rex*) and unspliced (*gag/pro-pol*) mRNAs, stabilizing them, and promoting their transport to the cytoplasm [62, 71] (Fig. 2.2).

### 2.2.3 Accessory Proteins: HBZ, p30, p12, p13, and p8

In contrast to Tax and Rex, HTLV-1 accessory genes *HBZ*, *p30*, *p12*, *p13*, and *p8* are not absolutely required for virus replication and for the immortalization of human primary T cells in vitro [31, 105, 149]. However, investigations using animal models to study HTLV-1 infection in vivo revealed that *HBZ*, *p30*, and *p12* are essential for HTLV-1 infection and replication in nonhuman primates but *p30* and *p12* were dispensable in rabbits [181]. Human T-cell lines immortalized with HTLV-1 molecular clones lacking *p30* or *p12* grow less efficiently than their wild-type counterpart clones and more dependent on the presence of interleukin-2 (IL-2) in the media [1, 131, 170].

#### 2.2.3.1 Viral Persistence and HTLV-1-Related Pathogenesis by HBZ

HBZ (HTLV-1 bZIP factor) is encoded by the minus strand of the HTLV-1 provirus and interacts with various host factors [3, 46, 125] (Fig. 2.1). The bZIP domain of HBZ is responsible for the interaction with the host bZIP factors, such as c-Jun, JunB, JunD [11, 172], CREB, CREB2 (ATF-4), CREM, ATF-1 [109], ATF-3 [53], and MafB [132]. The interaction mostly results in the suppression of transcriptional activity, including the Tax-mediated viral gene transcription from 5′ LTR, whereas the interaction with JunD activates transcription of target genes [172]. HBZ also enhances the TGFβ/Smad pathway, which is suppressed by Tax, through interaction with Smad2/3 and p300 [198], and then induces the expression of FoxP3 [89], a master regulatory molecule of regulatory T (Treg) cells. On the other hand, the transcriptional activity of Foxp3 is repressed by the interaction with HBZ [153]. As a result, HBZ increases the number of functionally impaired Treg cells and may lead to the development of malignancy derived from Treg cells.

Tax activates two types of NF-κB pathway, canonical and noncanonical (see the following section). p65 activation in the canonical pathway enhances the expression of CDK inhibitors p21 and p27, which cause the senescence of Tax-expressing cells. HBZ selectively inhibits the canonical NF-κB pathway by inhibiting DNA binding of p65 and promoting the degradation of p65 [199]. Thus, co-expression of HBZ with Tax delay or prevent the Tax-induced senescence, leading to cell proliferation.

Besides the functional modulation of various cellular transcription factors through protein-protein interaction, *HBZ* mRNA itself exerts a growth-promoting effect on T cells [152] (Fig. 2.1b). The first exon of the *HBZ* transcript corresponding to the R region of 3′ LTR, which forms an extensive stem-loop structure, is critical for this activity. Further details of how *HBZ* RNA promotes proliferation remain to be elucidated.

#### 2.2.3.2 Posttranscriptional Regulation of Viral and Cellular RNA by p30

p30 is a basic 241-amino acid protein encoded by the doubly spliced mRNA distinct from *tax/rex* mRNA (Fig. 2.1). p30 binds to the splice junction region of *tax/rex* mRNA and inhibits its nuclear export, thereby reducing the expression of Tax and Rex (Fig. 2.2). Conversely, Rex interacts with p30 and counteracts its activity to induce the expression of Tax/Rex proteins [8].

p30 expression activates the G2-M cell cycle checkpoint [29] and inhibits G1-S progression and homologous recombination (HR) repair to increase the genome instability through the protein-protein interaction with cyclin E/CDK2 and Nbs1/Rad50, respectively [13, 14]. Human T cells immortalized by a HTLV-1 proviral clone defective in p30 expression were more susceptible to apoptosis induced by camptothecin, a topoisomerase I inhibitor.

#### 2.2.3.3 Augmentation of Reactive Oxygen Production by p13

p13 is identical to the C-terminal 87 amino acids of p30 but encoded by a distinct singly spliced mono-cistronic mRNA (Fig. 2.1). A highly basic protein, p13, localizes mostly to mitochondria [28] and triggers an inward K+ and Ca+ current causing depolarization, activation of the electron transport chain, and augmentation of reactive oxygen species (ROS) production [16, 156] (Fig. 2.1b). Ectopic expression of p13 significantly reduces the incidence and growth rate of tumors arising from c-myc- and Ha-ras-co-transfected rat embryo fibroblasts [157]; therefore, low level of ROS production might help keep the infected cells benign through selectively killing the transformed HTLV-1 cells.

#### 2.2.3.4 Modulation of Signal Transduction and Immune Response by p12/p8

p12 is a highly hydrophobic membrane protein of 99 amino acids and localized in the endoplasmic reticulum (ER) and Golgi complex [33]. p12 increases intracellular $Ca^{2+}$ concentration by interacting with two ER resident proteins – calnexin and calreticulin – that regulate $Ca^{2+}$ release from the ER [33]. Increased concentration of $Ca^{2+}$ leads to the activation of calcineurin to dephosphorylate NFAT, thereby augmenting the transcription of genes such as IL-2 [2]. p12 also interacts with the beta and gamma c chain of the IL-2R and enhances the phosphorylation of STAT5 and its DNA binding [131]. Thus, p12 decreases the IL-2 requirement for T-cell proliferation and promotes cell proliferation (Fig. 2.1b).

In addition, p12 interacts with the major histocompatibility complex (MHC) class 1 heavy chain to inhibit its interaction with β2-microglobulin, thereby inducing the proteasome-dependent degradation of MHC class I [80]. The down-modulation of MHC class I reduces CTL-mediated killing of HTLV-1 infected cells. Furthermore, p12 also reduces expression of ICAM-1 and ICAM-2 to evade NK cells, which recognize cells lacking MHC class I molecule (Fig. 2.1b).

Proteolytic cleavage of p12 removes the ER retention motifs to generate the C-terminal product p8 [182]. p8 is localized to the T-cell membrane to induce lymphocyte function-associated antigen-1 (LFA-l)-mediated cell clustering, augmenting the number and length of conduits (filopodia-like membrane extensions) which are involved in HTLV-1 transmission as discussed later (Figs. 2.1b and 2.4).

## 2.3 Transmission

HTLV-l is primarily transmitted from infected mother to child through breastfeeding, while sexual contact and blood transfusion are additional routes of transmission [51]. Initial infection in vivo first requires interaction with oral, gastrointestinal, or cervical mucosa except infection through blood transfer. HTLV-1 infected cells can directly bypass a disrupted mucosa [143], while HTLV-1-infected macrophages could transmigrate through an intact epithelium as observed for human immunodeficiency virus (HIV) [168, 177] (Fig. 2.3a). On the other hand, viral particles produced by HTLV-1 infected T cells have been shown to cross the epithelium within an endosome from the apical to the basal

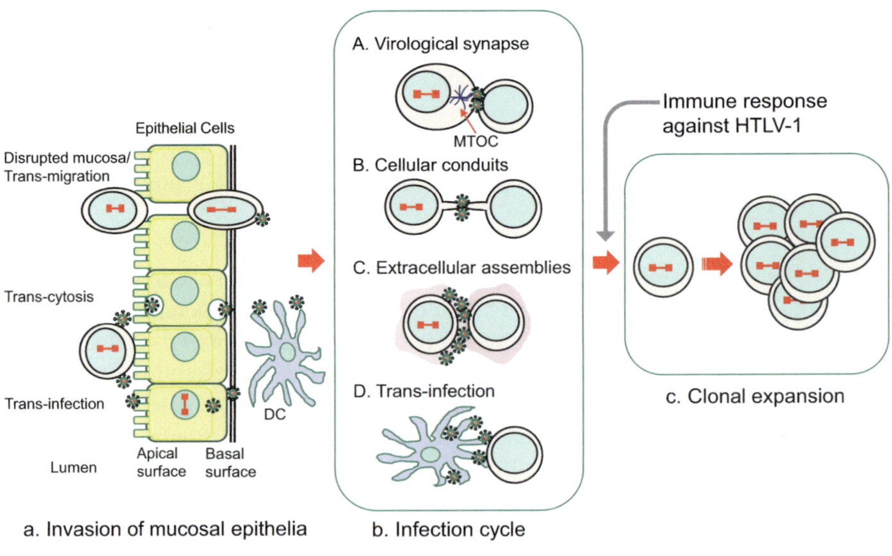


**Fig. 2.3** Transmission and expansion of HTLV-1. (**a**) Three different modes of mucosal invasion of HTLV-1. (**b**) Four different modes of cell-to-cell transmission of HTLV-1. (**c**) Clonal expansion mode of HTLV-1 replication

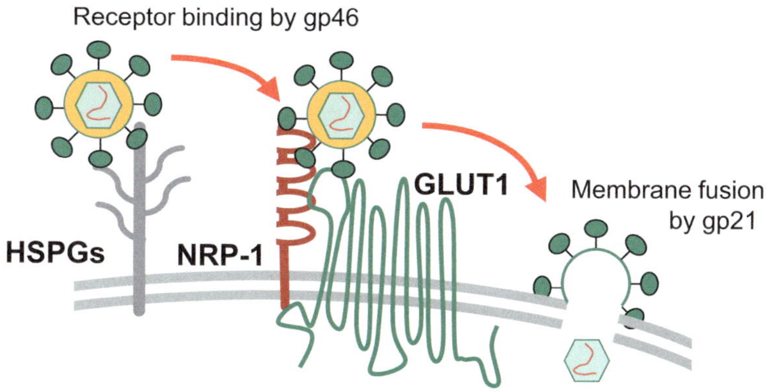


**Fig. 2.4** Model of HTLV-1 entry. Gp46 subunit of envelope protein attaches to heparan sulfate proteoglycans (*HSPGs*) on the target cell, which increases the local concentration of the viruses at the cell surface. Gp46 then binds to neuropilin-1 (*NRP-1*), and this binding induces a conformational change of the subunit that facilitates its interaction with glucose transporter 1 (*GLUT-1*). The formation of a ternary complex of gp46, NRP-1, and GLUT-1 induces a conformational change of gp21 that triggers the fusion of the viral and cell membranes

surface of an epithelial cell (transcytosis) [122]. Alternatively, HTLV-1 can also infect an epithelial cell and produce new virions that are then released from the basal surface [143, 195].

Having crossed the epithelial barrier, HTLV-1 infects mucosal immune cells directly or via APCs such as DCs or macrophages. APCs can either undergo infection or transfer membrane-bound extracellular virions to uninfected T cells (trans-infection) [83]. HTLV-1 predominantly infects CD4+ T cells but also targets other cell types such as CD8+ T and B lymphocytes, dendritic cells (DCs), monocytes, and macrophages [83, 101, 116].

HTLV-1 entry into susceptible cells begins with the binding of the HTLV-1 envelope glycoprotein (Env) to a viral receptor on the membrane of the host cell, and it is followed by the fusion of viral and cell membranes (Fig. 2.4). Efficient entry of HTLV-1 has been shown to involve three distinct molecules: heparin sulfate proteoglycans (HSPGs) and neuropilin 1 (NRP-1) for the initial binding to the cell and glucose transporter 1 (GLUT1) for entry [47, 82, 107, 120]. These molecules are ubiquitously expressed and may explain the wide range of target cells, but HTLV-l might differentially utilize these molecules in a cell type-dependent manner. In the current model, HTLV-1 Env first attaches to HSPGs on the target cell, which increases the local concentration of the viruses at the cell surface. HTLV-1 Env then binds to NRP-1, inducing a conformational change of Env that facilitates its interaction with GLUT-1. The ternary complex formation of Env, NRP-1, and GLUT-1 gives rise to an additional conformational change of Env that triggers the fusion of the viral and cell membranes.

HTLV-1 transmission usually occurs through cell-to-cell contact of HTLV-1-uninfected cells with HTLV-1-infected cells, and cell-free viruses are poorly infectious [30, 126]. Cell-to-cell transfer of HTLV-1 virions then potentially involves several nonexclusive mechanisms: a virological synapse [70, 119, 129], cellular conduits [182], or extracellular viral assemblies [81, 137] (Fig. 2.3b).

During cell-to-cell HTLV-1 transmission, the site of contact between an HTLV-1-infected cell and a target cell forms a special structure called the virological synapse (VS, named thus because of its similarity to the immunological synapse) [70] (Fig. 2.3b-A). VS formation involves polarization of the microtubule-organizing center (MTOC) near the site of cell-to-cell contact in the infected cells. ICAM-1 and Tax appear to play a role in polarization of the MTOC during cell-to-cell transmission.

HTLV-1 can also spread from an infected to an uninfected T cell by membrane extensions, which is referred to as cellular conduits [182] (Fig. 2.3b-B). HTLV-1 particles are concentrated at the point of contact between the HTLV-1-infected cell and the target cell.

Extracellular carbohydrate-rich assemblies attached to the surfaces of HTLV-l-infected cells contain infectious virions, and their removal prominently reduces cell-to-cell HTLV-1 transmission [137] (Fig. 2.3b-C). These virion-containing assemblies resemble bacterial biofilm in structure and composition and contain HSPGs, collagen, agrin, and galectin-3. When HTLV-1-infected T cells are exposed to uninfected T cells, these assemblies are quickly transferred to the target cell [137].

In addition to spreading between T cells, HTLV-1 can be transmitted from DCs to CD4+ T cells in two different ways, *cis*- and *trans*-infection. In *cis* mode of transmission, the DCs are infected, and then the de novo produced HTLV-1 is transferred to the T cells [83] (Fig. 2.3b-D). In the *trans*-infection, uninfected DCs capture and transmit the virus to T cells prior to becoming infected themselves [74].

## 2.4 Clonal Expansion and Immune Response

Soon after primary infection, HTLV-1 expands by reverse transcription of the viral RNA, integration of the provirus into the chromosome, expression of viral proteins, and budding of new virions (the infectious cycle, Fig. 2.3b). At this stage of infection, host restriction factors such as SAMHD1 [164], APOBEC3 [136], and miR-28-3p [7] have been shown to limit HTLV-1 infection.

An antiviral immune response is quickly initiated, and the efficacy of the infectious cycle is severely attenuated soon after infection. Then, HTLV-1 replicates through another mode of replication which involves mitotic division of a cell containing an integrated provirus (the clonal expansion, Fig. 2.3c). The limited variability in the HTLV-1 genome compared to HIV suggests a replication mode by cellular DNA polymerase rather than by error-prone viral reverse transcriptase in a major part of viral expansion. In fact, high-throughput sequencing of proviral integration sites reveal a high clonal stability over years [50].

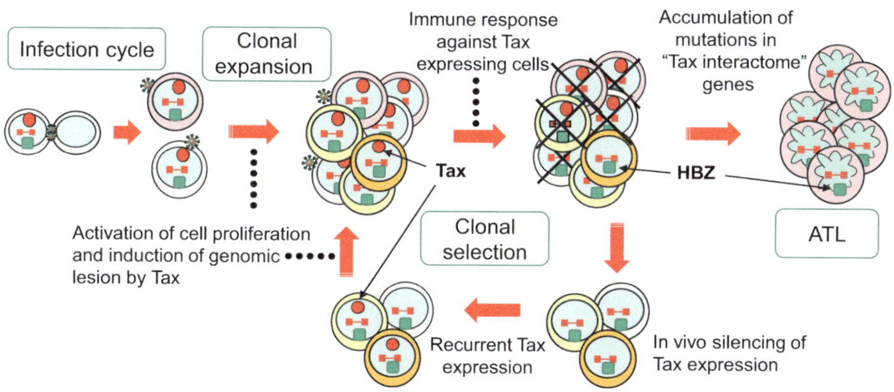


**Fig. 2.5** Model of clonal selection and ATL development. In early stage of infection, Tax and HBZ promote the proliferation of infected cells as well as the induction of genomic lesions (clonal expansion). Because of strong immunogenicity of Tax, Tax-expressing cells are rapidly eliminated. However, a substantial part of infected cells is escaped from the immune response due to the in vivo specific silencing mechanism of viral expression. Repetitive cycles of viral expression followed by transcriptional silencing lead to clonal selection and accumulation of mutations, finally in genes of Tax interactome, a network of molecules that Tax physically interacts with and/or deregulates, in ATL

On the other hand, clonal expansion and cell proliferation also require expression of viral factors such as Tax [19]. The in vivo proliferation of CD4+ T cells correlates with Tax expression [6]. Because Tax is a major target of CTLs [73, 84], Tax-expressing cells are rapidly eliminated (Fig. 2.5). However, transcription of the *tax* gene from the 5′ LTR is suppressed in vivo, and ex vivo culture of HTLV-1-infected cells elicits a rapid recovery of the tax gene expression [173], indicating a mechanism of inhibiting viral gene transcription in vivo [45, 56, 78]. Thus, repetitive cycles of viral expression followed by transcriptional silencing continuously challenge the immune response, thereby initiating inflammation and ultimately leading to HAM/TSP. Identification of integration sites by high-throughput sequencing shows that negative selection is predominant in chronic infection [50]. By favoring emergence of sporadic mutations in the cell genome, unrestrained proliferation also paves the way to malignant transformation and development of ATL [6, 91] (Fig. 2.5).

## 2.5 Leukemogenesis by Tax and HBZ

Among an array of viral factors, Tax and HBZ play a major role in leukemogenesis of HTLV-1 infected cells. Tax immortalizes human T cells in the presence of IL-2 and transforms rat fibroblasts and drives tumor formation in transgenic mouse models, supporting its oncogenic potential [52, 60, 133]. Mutation of the *tax* gene in recombinant HTLV-1 abrogates immortalization as well as persistent infection in rabbits [148].

Although HBZ is dispensable for the HTLV-1-mediated T-cell transformation in vitro, it plays an indispensable role in persistent viral infection in vivo [3]. In transgenic mouse model, HBZ expression in CD4 T cells induces chronic inflammation and T-cell lymphoma [153]. Furthermore, HBZ is constitutively expressed throughout HTLV-1 infection [91, 124, 180], whereas Tax expression is frequently suppressed or diminished in ATL cells [91, 98, 167], indicating the role of HBZ in maintaining the transformed phenotype [125]. Because of the strong immunogenicity of the Tax protein, these mechanisms can confer a selective advantage to HTLV-1-transformed T cells [73, 84, 86] (Fig. 2.5). In contrast, HBZ triggers a less efficient immunity that renders its persistent expression in vivo [64, 117].

An integrated genome analysis of a large number of ATL cases revealed that the driver mutations overlap significantly with the Tax interactome [19], a network of molecules that Tax physically interacts with and/or deregulates [91]. Thus, it seems that ATL cells still depend on deregulated Tax interactome molecules, even though Tax itself is no longer expressed in most ATL cases.

The modes of action of Tax and HBZ are remarkably pleiotropic and involve a variety of cell signaling pathways (CREB, NF-κB, and AKT, Fig. 2.2).

Tax inhibits tumor suppressors (p53 [147], Bcl11B [166], and TP53INP1 [192]) and activates cyclin-dependent kinases (CDKs) [55, 69, 134, 151], both of these mechanisms leading to accelerated cell proliferation. In addition, Tax induces genomic instability [20, 21, 23, 95], generating somatic alterations [121], and attenuates the Mad1 spindle assembly checkpoint protein, thereby promoting aneuploidy [79].

HBZ counteracts Tax-mediated viral and cellular pathway modulation (such as NF-κB, Akt, and CREB) and stimulates cell proliferation via apoptosis/senescence inhibition and cell cycle modulation [4, 152]. The interaction of HBZ with AP-1 factors (c-Jun, JunB, or MafB) results in the inhibition of their transcriptional activities and prevents the subsequent activation of AP-1-regulated genes [26, 67, 123].

### *2.5.1 Activation of NF-κB*

The NF-κB pathway is a key player in regulation of immunity and inflammation [161], and Tax activates the transcription factor NF-κB, thereby inducing the expression of several cellular genes. HTLV-1 carrying a mutant Tax that cannot activate NF-κB fails to immortalize human T cells in vitro [148]. Moreover, several NF-κB inhibitors induce apoptosis in HTLV-l-infected T cells. Thus, the NF-κB activity is crucial for the immortalization and the survival of HTLV-1 infected T cells.

By activating the NF-κB pathway, Tax upregulates antiapoptotic proteins: caspase-8 inhibitory protein c-FLIP [102, 135] and members of the Bcl-2 family

(Bcl-2, Bcl-xL, Mcl-1 and Blf-1) [115, 130, 163, 176], thereby supporting the proliferation and survival of HTLV-1-infected T cells. A variety of growth-promoting cytokines (such as IL-1, IL-6, TNF, and EGF) [88, 187] are also induced by Tax through the activation of NF-κB.

Conversely, NF-κB activation by Tax is associated with an upregulation of $p21^{WAF1/CIP1}$ and $p27^{KIP1}$, leading to cellular senescence [68, 200]. Instead, HBZ prevents Tax-induced senescence through downregulation of NF-κB [141, 200].

NF-κB is a family of transcription factors, and these factors are divided into two groups belonging to the canonical (NF-κB1/p50, p65, c-Rel) and the noncanonical (NF-κB2/p52, RelB, Bcl-3) pathways. Tax activates both pathways.

Through interacting with IKKγ/NEMO, a scaffold component of the IκB kinase (IKK) complex (IKKα/IKKβ/IKKγ), Tax activates the IKKβ to induce phosphorylation and degradation of IκBs (IκBα, IκBγ), allowing nuclear translocation of p50/p65 complex to activate transcription of NF-κB-responsive genes (canonical pathway) [58, 161]. Concurrently, the IKKα is activated to phosphorylate p65, which stimulates its transcriptional activation function.

Tax interaction with another IKK complex composed of IKKα and IKKγ, but not IKKβ, induces IKKα-dependent processing of p100 into p52 [58, 161] and the subsequent nuclear translocation of p52/RelB (noncanonical pathway). Knockdown of NF-κB2/p100 abrogates the Tax-induced transformation of CTLL-2 cell in vitro [63], and the knockout of NF-κB2/p100 gene attenuates the tumorigenesis in Tax transgenic mouse [41].

Although the constitutive activation of NF-κB pathway is crucial for the transformed phenotype of HTLV-1-infected T cells, ATL cells often lack the Tax expression due to deletions or epigenetic silencing of the 5′ LTR or mutations in Tax [66, 167]. The mechanisms of Tax-independent chronic activation of NF-κB remain poorly understood but may result from epigenetic alterations. Epigenetic downregulation of microRNA-31 (miR-31) in ATL promotes increased the expression of NIK (NF-κB-inducing kinase) that activates IKKα and noncanonical NF-κB pathway [189]. The expression of NIK is also enhanced by double-stranded RNA (dsRNA)-dependent protein kinase (PKR) that is activated by antisense transcripts at R region detected in all ATL cases [96].

### *2.5.2 Activation of the PI3K/AKT Pathway*

Tax promotes cell proliferation and survival through the activation of the phosphatidylinositol 3-kinase (PI3K)/Akt pathway [140]. Tax directly interacts with the p85α inhibitory subunit of PI3K, causing the release of the active p110α catalytic subunit [140]. Inhibition of Akt in HTLV-1-transformed cells decreases phosphorylated Bad and induces caspase-dependent apoptosis [77].

In contrast, HBZ inhibits Tax-dependent activation of the PI3K/Akt pathway and downstream antiapoptotic properties [160]. HBZ suppresses apoptosis by attenuating the function of FOXO3a and altering its localization [169].

### 2.5.3 Modulation of TGF-β/Smad and Wnt Signaling Pathways

Tax represses TGF-β signaling by blocking the association of Smad proteins with Smad-binding elements [108] and via c-Jun activation [5]. Conversely, HBZ interacts with Smad2/3 to enhance TGF-β/Smad transcriptional responses in a p300-dependent manner, improving transcription of different genes, such as the FOXP3 mediator of regulatory T cells [198]. This activation also results in the enhanced transcription of Wnt5a, a key protein of the noncanonical Wnt pathway. Knockdown of Wnt5a represses proliferation and migration of ATL cells, indicating the role of this pathway in HTLV-1-infected cell growth [113].

Tax interacts with DAPLE (dishevelled-associating protein with a high frequency of leucine residues) to activate the canonical Wnt pathway, whereas HBZ suppresses this activation by inhibiting DNA binding of TCF-1/LEF-1 transcription factors in the downstream.

### 2.5.4 Enhancement of S Phase Entry and Cell Cycle Progression

Through interaction with cyclins and CDKs, Tax interferes with cell cycle progression by several mechanisms. By stabilizing the cyclin D2/CDK4 complex and repressing cyclin-dependent kinase inhibitors (CKIs) such as members of INK4 family and KIP1, Tax enhances the phosphorylation of retinoblastoma protein (Rb) to free E2F1 that activates transcription of genes required for G1/S transition.

Tax also activates the cyclin D1 transcription via CREB pathway, thereby enhancing S phase entry of HTLV-1 infected cells, whereas HBZ interacts with CREB and inhibits transcription of cyclin D1 [114]. Early firing of late replication origins by Tax is associated with p300-dependent histone hyperacetylation, and interaction of Tax with the replicative helicase (minichromosome maintenance complex, MCM2-7) also accelerates S phase progression [20].

In contrast to Tax, HBZ modulates expression of cell division cycle 2 (CDC2) and cyclin E2 through interaction with activating transcription factor 3 (ATF3), thereby promoting proliferation of ATL cells [53]. Concomitantly, HBZ suppresses ATF3-induced p53 transcriptional activity. Moreover, the growth-promoting effect of *HBZ* mRNA on T cells is correlated with the enhanced transcription of E2F1 gene [152].

### 2.5.5 *Induction of Chromosomal Abnormality and DNA Damage*

The tumor-suppressor protein p53, the main factor that controls G1 checkpoint, is functionally inactivated in leukemic and HTLV-1 transformed cells [165]. NF-κB p65 subunit is critical for Tax-induced p53 inactivation [144] and wild-type p53-induced phosphatase 1 (Wip1) is involved in the inactivation [49, 196].

ATL cells are characterized by loss of spindle assembly checkpoint function [90] and aneuploidy [190]. Tax binding to Mad1 perturbs the organization of the spindle assembly and results in multinucleated cells [79]. Tax also interacts with the anaphase-promoting complex APC Cdc20, inducing the mitotic abnormalities in HTLV-1-infected cells [111].

Firing of supplementary origins of replication by Tax triggers replicative stress and genomic lesions, such as double-strand breaks (DSBs) [21, 23], which generate reactive oxygen species (ROS) [95]. Tax-associated DNA damages activate several phosphoproteins of the DDR pathway (H2AX, ATM, CHK1-2, P53, BRCA1), which in turn arrest the cell cycle transiently or lead to apoptosis and senescence. In the presence of DNA-damaging agents (e.g., UV irradiation), Tax inhibits the DDR machinery by sequestrating key signaling pathway components [15, 24, 35, 57, 138, 139]. Induction of genomic lesions and inhibition of the DDR leads to proliferation in presence of DNA mutations, potentially to leukemogenesis.

HBZ also induces DNA lesions through activation of miR-17 and miR-21 and downregulation of the DNA damage factor OBFC2A [183] and deregulates the cellular responses to DNA damage by inhibiting the activity of growth arrest and DNA damage gene 34 (GADD34) [128].

In addition, Tax has negative effects on DNA repair pathways. Downregulation of β-polymerase transcription by Tax [76] leads to the inhibition of base excision repair (BER) [142]. Tax interferes with nucleotide excision repair (NER) by activating PCNA [87, 110] and suppresses nonhomologous end joining (NHEJ) by repressing Ku80 gene transcription and also by interacting with Ku80 protein [34, 118], while DSBs are preferentially repaired by error-prone NHEJ in Tax-expressing cells [12].

## 2.6 Animal Model

To evaluate viral pathogenesis and elucidate the function of viral products in vivo, a variety of animal models have been established [9, 32, 39, 45, 60, 99, 153, 184]. The Tax transgenic mouse, which expresses Tax under the control of the Lck promoter, results in characteristic ATL-like phenotypes [60]. The HBZ transgenic mouse, which expresses HBZ under the control of a CD4-specific promoter/enhancer/silencer, develops lymphomas characterized by induction of Foxp3 in CD4 T cells, similar to leukemic cells in ATL patients [153].

In addition to transgenic mouse models, a number of HTLV-1-infected small-animal models have provided valuable findings regarding virus-host interactions; however, they are unable to fully recapitulate pathological conditions resembling ATL, likely due to the low efficiency of HTLV-1 infection [93, 106].

As immune responses against HTLV-1 play a pivotal role in controlling the proliferation or selection of HTLV-1-infected T-cell clones in vivo [59, 85], animal models of ATL that induce more humanlike HTLV-1-specific immune responses are required for analysis of the development of ATL. Humanized mice are highly susceptible to infection with human lymphotropic viruses, such as EBV, HIV-1, and HTLV-1, and are able to recapitulate specific disorders and human immune responses [184, 185, 188]. HTLV-1 infection of humanized mouse, which is produced by the intra-bone marrow transplantation of human hematopoietic stem cells, displayed distinct ATL-like symptoms, including hepatosplenomegaly, hypercytokinemia, oligoclonal proliferation of HTLV-1-infected T cells, and the appearance of flower cells [171]. Furthermore, HTLV-1-specific immunity was induced.

## 2.7 Perspective

Since the discovery of HTLV-1, extensive studies have revealed a complex network of interactions between viral genes and host factors. This network controls the expression of viral genes and facilitates persistent infection by allowing evasion of the host immune response and promoting the proliferation of infected cells.

Recent findings from the integrated molecular study of ATL genome provide a strong evidence for the notion that the aberrant growth-promoting activities attributed to Tax function are taken over by mutations in genes belonging to the Tax interactome [91]. Knowledge of the genes and the mutations will guide the development of new diagnostics and therapeutics for ATL.

As the incident rate of mutations correlates with the number of infected cells and, probably, with Tax expression during persistent infection, it is important to control the viral expression and the clonal expansion of infected cells in vivo to suppress the onset of ATL. Therefore, further analysis with suitable animal model of HTLV-1 infection, in which anti-HTLV-1 immune response is established, should provide vital information for developing antiviral and/or preventive therapy.

## References

1. Albrecht B, Collins ND, Burniston MT, Nisbet JW, Ratner L, Green PL, Lairmore MD. Human T-lymphotropic virus type 1 open reading frame I p12(I) is required for efficient viral infectivity in primary lymphocytes. J Virol. 2000;74:9828–35.

2. Albrecht B, D'Souza CD, Ding W, Tridandapani S, Coggeshall KM, Lairmore MD. Activation of nuclear factor of activated T cells by human T-lymphotropic virus type 1 accessory protein p12(I). J Virol. 2002;76:3493–501. doi:10.1128/JVI.76.7.3493-3501.2002.
3. Arnold J. Enhancement of infectivity and persistence in vivo by HBZ, a natural antisense coded protein of HTLV-1. Blood. 2006;107:3976–82. doi:10.1182/blood-2005-11-4551.
4. Arnold J, Zimmerman B, Li M, Lairmore MD, Green PL. Human T-cell leukemia virus type-1 antisense-encoded gene, Hbz, promotes T-lymphocyte proliferation. Blood. 2008;112:3788–97. doi:10.1182/blood-2008-04-154286.
5. Arnulf B, Villemain A, Nicot C, Mordelet E, Charneau P, Kersual J, Zermati Y, Mauviel A, Bazarbachi A, Hermine O. Human T-cell lymphotropic virus oncoprotein Tax represses TGF-beta 1 signaling in human T cells via c-Jun activation: a potential mechanism of HTLV-I leukemogenesis. Blood. 2002;100:4129–38. doi:10.1182/blood-2001-12-0372.
6. Asquith B, Zhang Y, Mosley AJ, de Lara CM, Wallace DL, Worth A, Kaftantzi L, Meekings K, Griffin GE, Tanaka Y, Tough DF, Beverley PC, Taylor GP, Macallan DC, Bangham CRM. In vivo T lymphocyte dynamics in humans and the impact of human T-lymphotropic virus 1 infection. Proc Natl Acad Sci U S A. 2007;104:8035–40. doi:10.1073/pnas.0608832104.
7. Bai XT, Nicot C. miR-28-3p is a cellular restriction factor that inhibits human T cell leukemia virus, type 1 (HTLV-1) replication and virus infection. J Biol Chem. 2015;290:5381–90. doi:10.1074/jbc.M114.626325.
8. Bai XT, Sinha-Datta U, Ko NL, Bellon M, Nicot C. Nuclear export and expression of human T-cell leukemia virus type 1 tax/rex mRNA are RxRE/Rex dependent. J Virol. 2012;86:4559–65. doi:10.1128/JVI.06361-11.
9. Banerjee P, Tripp A, Lairmore MD, Crawford L, Sieburg M, Ramos JC, Harrington W, Beilke MA, Feuer G. Adult T-cell leukemia/lymphoma development in HTLV-1-infected humanized SCID mice. Blood. 2010;115:2640–8. doi:10.1182/blood-2009-10-246959.
10. Bantignies F, Rousset R, Desbois C, Jalinot P. Genetic characterization of transactivation of the human T-cell leukemia virus type 1 promoter: binding of tax to tax -responsive element 1 is mediated by the cyclic AMP-responsive members of the CREB/ATF family of transcription factors. Mol Cell Biol. 1996;16:2174–82.
11. Basbous J, Arpin C, Gaudray G, Piechaczyk M, Devaux C, Mesnard J-M. The HBZ factor of human T-cell leukemia virus type I dimerizes with transcription factors JunB and c-Jun and modulates their transcriptional activity. J Biol Chem. 2003;278:43620–7. doi:10.1074/jbc.M307275200.
12. Baydoun HH, Bai XT, Shelton S, Nicot C. HTLV-I tax increases genetic instability by inducing DNA double strand breaks during DNA replication and switching repair to NHEJ. PLoS ONE. 2012;7:e42226. doi:10.1371/journal.pone.0042226.
13. Baydoun HH, Pancewicz J, Bai X, Nicot C. HTLV-I p30 inhibits multiple S phase entry checkpoints, decreases cyclin E-CDK2 interactions and delays cell cycle progression. Mol Cancer. 2010;9:302. doi:10.1186/1476-4598-9-302.
14. Baydoun HH, Pancewicz J, Nicot C. Human T-lymphotropic type 1 virus p30 inhibits homologous recombination and favors unfaithful DNA repair. Blood. 2011;117:5897–906. doi:10.1182/blood-2010-08-304600.
15. Belgnaoui SM, Fryrear KA, Nyalwidhe JO, Guo X, Semmes OJ. The viral oncoprotein tax sequesters DNA damage response factors by tethering MDC1 to chromatin. J Biol Chem. 2010;285:32897–905. doi:10.1074/jbc.M110.146373.
16. Biasiotto R, Aguiari P, Rizzuto R, Pinton P, D'Agostino DM, Ciminale V. The p13 protein of human T cell leukemia virus type 1 (HTLV-1) modulates mitochondrial membrane potential and calcium uptake. Biochim Biophys Acta. 2010;1797:945–51. doi:10.1016/j.bbabio.2010.02.023.
17. Bogerd HP, Huckaby GL, Ahmed YF, Hanly SM, Greene WC. The type I human T-cell leukemia virus (HTLV-I) Rex trans-activator binds directly to the HTLV-I Rex and the type

1 human immunodeficiency virus Rev RNA response elements. Proc Natl Acad Sci U S A. 1991;88:5704–8.
18. Bogerd HP, Tiley LS, Cullen BR. Specific binding of the human T-cell leukemia virus type I Rex protein to a short RNA sequence located within the Rex-response element. J Virol. 1992;66:7572–5.
19. Boxus M, Twizere J-C, Legros S, Dewulf J-F, Kettmann R, Willems L. The HTLV-1 Tax interactome. Retrovirology. 2008;5:76. doi:10.1186/1742-4690-5-76.
20. Boxus M, Twizere J-C, Legros S, Kettmann R, Willems L. Interaction of HTLV-1 Tax with minichromosome maintenance proteins accelerates the replication timing program. Blood. 2012;119:151–60. doi:10.1182/blood-2011-05-356790.
21. Boxus M, Willems L. How the DNA damage response determines the fate of HTLV-1 Tax-expressing cells. Retrovirology. 2012;9:2. doi:10.1186/1742-4690-9-2.
22. Brady J, Jeang KT, Duvall J, Khoury G. Identification of p40x-responsive regulatory sequences within the human T-cell leukemia virus type I long terminal repeat. J Virol. 1987;61:2175–81.
23. Chaib-Mezrag H, Lemaçon D, Fontaine H, Bellon M, Bai XT, Drac M, Coquelle A, Nicot C. Tax impairs DNA replication forks and increases DNA breaks in specific oncogenic genome regions. Mol Cancer. 2014;13:205. doi:10.1186/1476-4598-13-205.
24. Chandhasin C, Ducu RI, Berkovich E, Kastan MB, Marriott SJ. Human T-cell leukemia virus type 1 tax attenuates the ATM-mediated cellular DNA damage response. J Virol. 2008;82:6952–61. doi:10.1128/JVI.02331-07.
25. Ciminale V, Pavlakis GN, Derse D, Cunningham CP, Felber BK. Complex splicing in the human T-cell leukemia virus (HTLV) family of retroviruses: novel mRNAs and proteins produced by HTLV type I. J Virol. 1992;66:1737–45.
26. Clerc I, Hivin P, Rubbo P-A, Lemasson I, Barbeau B, Mesnard J-M. Propensity for HBZ-SP1 isoform of HTLV-I to inhibit c-Jun activity correlates with sequestration of c-Jun into nuclear bodies rather than inhibition of its DNA-binding activity. Virology. 2009;391:195–202. doi:10.1016/j.virol.2009.06.027.
27. Conkright MD, Canettieri G, Screaton R, Guzmán E, Miraglia L, Hogenesch JB, Montminy M. TORCs: transducers of regulated CREB activity. Mol Cell. 2003;12:413–23.
28. D'Agostino DM, Silic-Benussi M, Hiraragi H, Lairmore MD, Ciminale V. The human T-cell leukemia virus type 1 p13II protein: effects on mitochondrial function and cell growth. Cell Death Differ. 2005;12(Suppl 1):905–15. doi:10.1038/sj.cdd.4401576.
29. Datta A, Silverman L, Phipps AJ, Hiraragi H, Ratner L, Lairmore MD. Human T-lymphotropic virus type-1 p30 alters cell cycle G2 regulation of T lymphocytes to enhance cell survival. Retrovirology. 2007;4:49. doi:10.1186/1742-4690-4-49.
30. Derse D, Hill SA, Lloyd PA, Chung H, Morse BA. Examining human T-cell leukemia virus type 1 infection and replication by cell-free infection with recombinant virus vectors. J Virol. 2001;75:8461–8. doi:10.1128/JVI.75.18.8461-8468.2001.
31. Derse D, Mikovits J, Ruscetti F. X-I and X-II open reading frames of HTLV-I are not required for virus replication or for immortalization of primary T-cells in vitro. Virology. 1997;237:123–8. doi:10.1006/viro.1997.8781.
32. Dewan MZ, Terashima K, Taruishi M, Hasegawa H, Ito M, Tanaka Y, Mori N, Sata T, Koyanagi Y, Maeda M, Kubuki Y, Okayama A, Fujii M, Yamamoto N. Rapid tumor formation of human T-cell leukemia virus type 1-infected cell lines in novel NOD-SCID/gammac(null) mice: suppression by an inhibitor against NF-kappaB. J Virol. 2003;77:5286–94. doi:10.1128/JVI.77.9.5286-5294.2003.
33. Ding W, Albrecht B, Luo R, Zhang W, Stanley JR, Newbound GC, Lairmore MD. Endoplasmic reticulum and cis-Golgi localization of human T-lymphotropic virus type 1 p12(I): association with calreticulin and calnexin. J Virol. 2001;75:7672–82. doi:10.1128/JVI.75.16.7672-7682.2001.
34. Ducu RI, Dayaram T, Marriott SJ. The HTLV-1 Tax oncoprotein represses Ku80 gene expression. Virology. 2011;416:1–8. doi:10.1016/j.virol.2011.04.012.

35. Durkin SS, Guo X, Fryrear KA, Mihaylova VT, Gupta SK, Belgnaoui SM, Haoudi A, Kupfer GM, Semmes OJ. HTLV-1 Tax oncoprotein subverts the cellular DNA damage response via binding to DNA-dependent protein kinase. J Biol Chem. 2008;283:36311–20. doi:10.1074/jbc.M804931200.
36. Ellermann V, Bang O. Experimentelle Leukämie bei Hühnerm. Zentralbl Bakteriol Parasitenkd Infectionskr Hyg Abt Orig. 1908;46:595–609.
37. Felber BK, Paskalis H, Kleinman-Ewing C, Wong-Staal F, Pavlakis GN. The pX protein of HTLV-I is a transcriptional activator of its long terminal repeats. Science. 1985;229:675–9.
38. Feuer G, Chen IS. Mechanisms of human T-cell leukemia virus-induced leukemogenesis. Biochim Biophys Acta. 1992;1114:223–33.
39. Feuer G, Zack JA, Harrington WJ, Valderama R, Rosenblatt JD, Wachsman W, Baird SM, Chen IS. Establishment of human T-cell leukemia virus type I T-cell lymphomas in severe combined immunodeficient mice. Blood. 1993;82:722–31.
40. Franklin AA, Kubik MF, Uittenbogaard MN, Brauweiler A, Utaisincharoen P, Matthews MA, Dynan WS, Hoeffler JP, Nyborg JK. Transactivation by the human T-cell leukemia virus Tax protein is mediated through enhanced binding of activating transcription factor-2 (ATF-2) ATF-2 response and cAMP element-binding protein (CREB). J Biol Chem. 1993;268:21225–31.
41. Fu J, Qu Z, Yan P, Ishikawa C, Aqeilan RI, Rabson AB, Xiao G. The tumor suppressor gene WWOX links the canonical and noncanonical NF-κB pathways in HTLV-I Tax-mediated tumorigenesis. Blood. 2011;117:1652–61. doi:10.1182/blood-2010-08-303073.
42. Fujisawa J, Seiki M, Sato M, Yoshida M. A transcriptional enhancer sequence of HTLV-I is responsible for trans-activation mediated by p40 chi HTLV-I. EMBO J. 1986;5:713–8.
43. Fujisawa J, Toita M, Yoshida M. A unique enhancer element for the trans activator (p40tax) of human T-cell leukemia virus type I that is distinct from cyclic AMP- and 12-O-tetradecanoylphorbol-13-acetate-responsive elements. J Virol. 1989;63:3234–9.
44. Fujisawa J, Toita M, Yoshimura T, Yoshida M. The indirect association of human T-cell leukemia virus tax protein with DNA results in transcriptional activation. J Virol. 1991;65:4525–8.
45. Furuta RA, Sugiura K, Kawakita S, Inada T, Ikehara S, Matsuda T, Fujisawa J-I. Mouse model for the equilibration interaction between the host immune system and human T-cell leukemia virus type 1 gene expression. J Virol. 2002;76:2703–13. doi:10.1128/JVI.76.6.2703-2713.2002.
46. Gaudray G, Gachon F, Basbous J, Biard-Piechaczyk M, Devaux C, Mesnard J-M. The complementary strand of the human T-cell leukemia virus type 1 RNA genome encodes a bZIP transcription factor that down-regulates viral transcription. J Virol. 2002;76:12813–22. doi:10.1128/JVI.76.24.12813-12822.2002.
47. Ghez D, Lepelletier Y, Lambert S, Fourneau J-M, Blot V, Janvier S, Arnulf B, van Endert PM, Heveker N, Pique C, Hermine O. Neuropilin-1 is involved in human T-cell lymphotropic virus type 1 entry. J Virol. 2006;80:6844–54. doi:10.1128/JVI.02719-05.
48. Giam CZ, Xu YL. HTLV-I tax gene product activates transcription via pre-existing cellular factors and cAMP responsive element. J Biol Chem. 1989;264:15236–41.
49. Gillet N, Carpentier A, Barez P-Y, Willems L. WIP1 deficiency inhibits HTLV-1 Tax oncogenesis: novel therapeutic prospects for treatment of ATL? Retrovirology. 2012;9:115. doi:10.1186/1742-4690-9-115.
50. Gillet NA, Malani N, Melamed A, Gormley N, Carter R, Bentley D, Berry C, Bushman FD, Taylor GP, Bangham CRM. The host genomic environment of the provirus determines the abundance of HTLV-1-infected T-cell clones. Blood. 2011;117:3113–22. doi:10.1182/blood-2010-10-312926.
51. Gonçalves DU, Proietti FA, Ribas JGR, Araújo MG, Pinheiro SR, Guedes AC, Carneiro-Proietti ABF. Epidemiology, treatment, and prevention of human T-cell leukemia virus type 1-associated diseases. Clin Microbiol Rev. 2010;23:577–89. doi:10.1128/CMR.00063-09.

52. Grossman WJ, Kimata JT, Wong FH, Zutter M, Ley TJ, Ratner L. Development of leukemia in mice transgenic for the tax gene of human T-cell leukemia virus type I. Proc Natl Acad Sci U S A. 1995;92:1057–61.
53. Hagiya K, Yasunaga J-I, Satou Y, Ohshima K, Matsuoka M. ATF3, an HTLV-1 bZip factor binding protein, promotes proliferation of adult T-cell leukemia cells. Retrovirology. 2011;8:19. doi:10.1186/1742-4690-8-19.
54. Hakata Y, Umemoto T, Matsushita S, Shida H. Involvement of human CRM1 (exportin 1) in the export and multimerization of the Rex protein of human T-cell leukemia virus type 1. J Virol. 1998;72:6602–7.
55. Haller K, Wu Y, Derow E, Schmitt I, Jeang K-T, Grassmann R. Physical interaction of human T-cell leukemia virus type 1 Tax with cyclin-dependent kinase 4 stimulates the phosphorylation of retinoblastoma protein. Mol Cell Biol. 2002;22:3327–38. doi:10.1128/MCB.22.10.3327-3338.2002.
56. Hanon E, Hall S, Taylor GP, Saito M, Davis R, Tanaka Y, Usuku K, Osame M, Weber JN, Bangham CR. Abundant tax protein expression in CD4+ T cells infected with human T-cell lymphotropic virus type I (HTLV-I) is prevented by cytotoxic T lymphocytes. Blood. 2000;95:1386–92.
57. Haoudi A, Semmes OJ. The HTLV-1 tax oncoprotein attenuates DNA damage induced G1 arrest and enhances apoptosis in p53 null cells. Virology. 2003;305:229–39.
58. Harhaj EW, Harhaj NS. Mechanisms of persistent NF-kappaB activation by HTLV-I tax. IUBMB Life. 2005;57:83–91. doi:10.1080/15216540500078715.
59. Hasegawa A, Ohashi T, Hanabuchi S, Kato H, Takemura F, Masuda T, Kannagi M. Expansion of human T-cell leukemia virus type 1 (HTLV-1) reservoir in orally infected rats: inverse correlation with HTLV-1-specific cellular immune response. J Virol. 2003;77:2956–63.
60. Hasegawa H, Sawa H, Lewis MJ, Orba Y, Sheehy N, Yamamoto Y, Ichinohe T, Tsunetsugu-Yokota Y, Katano H, Takahashi H, Matsuda J, Sata T, Kurata T, Nagashima K, Hall WW. - Thymus-derived leukemia-lymphoma in mice transgenic for the Tax gene of human T-lymphotropic virus type I. Nat Med. 2006;12:466–72. doi:10.1038/nm1389.
61. Hattori S, Kiyokawa T, Imagawa K, Shimizu F, Hashimura E, Seiki M, Yoshida M. Identification of gag and env gene products of human T-cell leukemia virus (HTLV). Virology. 1984;136:338–47.
62. Hidaka M, Inoue J, Yoshida M, Seiki M. Post-transcriptional regulator (rex) of HTLV-1 initiates expression of viral structural proteins but suppresses expression of regulatory proteins. EMBO J. 1988;7:519–23.
63. Higuchi M, Tsubata C, Kondo R, Yoshida S, Takahashi M, Oie M, Tanaka Y, Mahieux R, Matsuoka M, Fujii M. Cooperation of NF-kappaB2/p100 activation and the PDZ domain binding motif signal in human T-cell leukemia virus type 1 (HTLV-1) Tax1 but not HTLV-2 Tax2 is crucial for interleukin-2-independent growth transformation of a T-cell line. J Virol. 2007;81:11900–7. doi:10.1128/JVI.00532-07.
64. Hilburn S, Rowan A, Demontis M-A, Macnamara A, Asquith B, Bangham CRM, Taylor GP. In vivo expression of human T-lymphotropic virus type 1 basic leucine-zipper protein generates specific CD8+ and CD4+ T-lymphocyte responses that correlate with clinical outcome. J Infect Dis. 2011;203:529–36. doi:10.1093/infdis/jiq078.
65. Hinuma Y, Nagata K, Hanaoka M, Nakai M, Matsumoto T, Kinoshita KI, Shirakawa S, Miyoshi I. Adult T-cell leukemia: antigen in an ATL cell line and detection of antibodies to the antigen in human sera. Proc Natl Acad Sci U S A. 1981;78:6476–80.
66. Hironaka N, Mochida K, Mori N, Maeda M, Yamamoto N, Yamaoka S. Tax-independent constitutive IkappaB kinase activation in adult T-cell leukemia cells. Neoplasia. 2004;6:266–78. doi:10.1593/neo.3388.
67. Hivin P, Basbous J, Raymond F, Henaff D, Arpin-André C, Robert-Hebmann V, Barbeau B, Mesnard J-M. The HBZ-SP1 isoform of human T-cell leukemia virus type I represses JunB

activity by sequestration into nuclear bodies. Retrovirology. 2007;4:14. doi:10.1186/1742-4690-4-14.
68. Ho Y-K, Zhi H, DeBiaso D, Philip S, Shih H-M, Giam C-Z. HTLV-1 tax-induced rapid senescence is driven by the transcriptional activity of NF-κB and depends on chronically activated IKKα and p65/RelA. J Virol. 2012;86:9474–83. doi:10.1128/JVI.00158-12.
69. Huang Y, Ohtani K, Iwanaga R, Matsumura Y, Nakamura M. Direct trans-activation of the human cyclin D2 gene by the oncogene product Tax of human T-cell leukemia virus type I. Oncogene. 2001;20:1094–102. doi:10.1038/sj.onc.1204198.
70. Igakura T, Stinchcombe JC, Goon PKC, Taylor GP, Weber JN, Griffiths GM, Tanaka Y, Osame M, Bangham CRM. Spread of HTLV-I between lymphocytes by virus-induced polarization of the cytoskeleton. Science. 2003;299:1713–6. doi:10.1126/science.1080115.
71. Inoue J, Itoh M, Akizawa T, Toyoshima H, Yoshida M. HTLV-1 Rex protein accumulates unspliced RNA in the nucleus as well as in cytoplasm. Oncogene. 1991;6:1753–7.
72. Iourgenko V, Zhang W, Mickanin C, Daly I, Jiang C, Hexham JM, Orth AP, Miraglia L, Meltzer J, Garza D, Chirn G-W, McWhinnie E, Cohen D, Skelton J, Terry R, Yu Y, Bodian D, Buxton FP, Zhu J, Song C, Labow MA. Identification of a family of cAMP response element-binding protein coactivators by genome-scale functional analysis in mammalian cells. Proc Natl Acad Sci U S A. 2003;100:12147–52. doi:10.1073/pnas.1932773100.
73. Jacobson S, Shida H, McFarlin DE, Fauci AS, Koenig S. Circulating CD8+ cytotoxic T lymphocytes specific for HTLV-I pX in patients with HTLV-I associated neurological disease. Nature. 1990;348:245–8. doi:10.1038/348245a0.
74. Jain P, Manuel SL, Khan ZK, Ahuja J, Quann K, Wigdahl B. DC-SIGN mediates cell-free infection and transmission of human T-cell lymphotropic virus type 1 by dendritic cells. J Virol. 2009;83:10908–21. doi:10.1128/JVI.01054-09.
75. Jeang KT, Boros I, Brady J, Radonovich M, Khoury G. Characterization of cellular factors that interact with the human T-cell leukemia virus type I p40x-responsive 21-base-pair sequence. J Virol. 1988;62:4499–509.
76. Jeang KT, Widen SG, Semmes OJ, Wilson SH. HTLV-I trans-activator protein, tax, is a trans-repressor of the human beta-polymerase gene. Science. 1990;247:1082–4.
77. Jeong S-J, Dasgupta A, Jung K-J, Um J-H, Burke A, Park HU, Brady JN. PI3K/AKT inhibition induces caspase-dependent apoptosis in HTLV-1-transformed cells. Virology. 2008;370:264–72. doi:10.1016/j.virol.2007.09.003.
78. Jiang S, Inada T, Tanaka M, Furuta RA, Shingu K, Fujisawa J-I. Involvement of TORC2, a CREB co-activator, in the in vivo-specific transcriptional control of HTLV-1. Retrovirology. 2009;6:73. doi:10.1186/1742-4690-6-73.
79. Jin DY, Spencer F, Jeang KT. Human T cell leukemia virus type 1 oncoprotein Tax targets the human mitotic checkpoint protein MAD1. Cell. 1998;93:81–91.
80. Johnson JM, Nicot C, Fullen J, Ciminale V, Casareto L, Mulloy JC, Jacobson S, Franchini G. Free major histocompatibility complex class I heavy chain is preferentially targeted for degradation by human T-cell leukemia/lymphotropic virus type 1 p12(I) protein. J Virol. 2001;75:6086–94. doi:10.1128/JVI.75.13.6086-6094.2001.
81. Jones KS, Green PL. Cloaked virus slips between cells. Nat Med. 2010;16:25–7. doi:10.1038/nm0110-25.
82. Jones KS, Petrow-Sadowski C, Bertolette DC, Huang Y, Ruscetti FW. Heparan sulfate proteoglycans mediate attachment and entry of human T-cell leukemia virus type 1 virions into CD4+ T cells. J Virol. 2005;79:12692–702. doi:10.1128/JVI.79.20.12692-12702.2005.
83. Jones KS, Petrow-Sadowski C, Huang YK, Bertolette DC, Ruscetti FW. Cell-free HTLV-1 infects dendritic cells leading to transmission and transformation of CD4(+) T cells. Nat Med. 2008;14:429–36. doi:10.1038/nm1745.
84. Kannagi M, Harada S, Maruyama I, Inoko H, Igarashi H, Kuwashima G, Sato S, Morita M, Kidokoro M, Sugimoto M. Predominant recognition of human T cell leukemia virus type I (HTLV-I) pX gene products by human CD8+ cytotoxic T cells directed against HTLV-I-infected cells. Int Immunol. 1991;3:761–7.

85. Kannagi M, Hasegawa A, Kinpara S, Shimizu Y, Takamori A, Utsunomiya A. Double control systems for human T-cell leukemia virus type 1 by innate and acquired immunity. Cancer Sci. 2011;102:670–6. doi:10.1111/j.1349-7006.2011.01862.x.
86. Kannagi M, Matsushita S, Harada S. Expression of the target antigen for cytotoxic T lymphocytes on adult T-cell-leukemia cells. Int J Cancer. 1993;54:582–8.
87. Kao SY, Marriott SJ. Disruption of nucleotide excision repair by the human T-cell leukemia virus type 1 Tax protein. J Virol. 1999;73:4299–304.
88. Karin M. NF-kappaB as a critical link between inflammation and cancer. Cold Spring Harb Perspect Biol. 2009;1:a000141–1. doi:10.1101/cshperspect.a000141.
89. Karube K, Ohshima K, Tsuchiya T, Yamaguchi T, Kawano R, Suzumiya J, Utsunomiya A, Harada M, Kikuchi M. Expression of FoxP3, a key molecule in CD4CD25 regulatory T cells, in adult T-cell leukaemia/lymphoma cells. Br J Haematol. 2004;126:81–4. doi:10.1111/j.1365-2141.2004.04999.x.
90. Kasai T, Iwanaga Y, Iha H, Jeang K-T. Prevalent loss of mitotic spindle checkpoint in adult T-cell leukemia confers resistance to microtubule inhibitors. J Biol Chem. 2002;277:5187–93. doi:10.1074/jbc.M110295200.
91. Kataoka K, Nagata Y, Kitanaka A, Shiraishi Y, Shimamura T, Yasunaga J-I, Totoki Y, Chiba K, Sato-Otsubo A, Nagae G, Ishii R, Muto S, Kotani S, Watatani Y, Takeda J, Sanada M, Tanaka H, Suzuki H, Sato Y, Shiozawa Y, Yoshizato T, Yoshida K, Makishima H, Iwanaga M, Ma G, Nosaka K, Hishizawa M, Itonaga H, Imaizumi Y, Munakata W, Ogasawara H, Sato T, Sasai K, Muramoto K, Penova M, Kawaguchi T, Nakamura H, Hama N, Shide K, Kubuki Y, Hidaka T, Kameda T, Nakamaki T, Ishiyama K, Miyawaki S, Yoon S-S, Tobinai K, Miyazaki Y, Takaori-Kondo A, Matsuda F, Takeuchi K, Nureki O, Aburatani H, Watanabe T, Shibata T, Matsuoka M, Miyano S, Shimoda K, Ogawa S. Integrated molecular analysis of adult T cell leukemia/lymphoma. Nat Genet. 2015;47:1304–15. doi:10.1038/ng.3415.
92. Katz RA, Skalka AM. Generation of diversity in retroviruses. Annu Rev Genet. 1990;24:409–45. doi:10.1146/annurev.ge.24.120190.002205.
93. Kazanji M. HTLV Type 1 infection in squirrel monkeys (*Saimiri sciureus*): a promising animal model for HTLV type 1 human infection. AIDS Res Hum Retrovir. 2000;16:1741–6. doi:10.1089/08892220050193245.
94. Kim Y-M, Ramírez JA, Mick JE, Giebler HA, Yan J-P, Nyborg JK. Molecular characterization of the Tax-containing HTLV-1 enhancer complex reveals a prominent role for CREB phosphorylation in Tax transactivation. J Biol Chem. 2007;282:18750–7. doi:10.1074/jbc.M700391200.
95. Kinjo T, Ham-Terhune J, Peloponese J-M, Jeang K-T. Induction of reactive oxygen species by human T-cell leukemia virus type 1 tax correlates with DNA damage and expression of cellular senescence marker. J Virol. 2010;84:5431–7. doi:10.1128/JVI.02460-09.
96. Kinpara S, Ito S, Takahata T, Saitoh Y, Hasegawa A, Kijiyama M, Utsunomiya A, Masuda M, Miyazaki Y, Matsuoka M, Nakamura M, Yamaoka S, Masuda T, Kannagi M. Involvement of double-stranded RNA-dependent protein kinase and antisense viral RNA in the constitutive NFκB activation in adult T-cell leukemia/lymphoma cells. Leukemia. 2015;29:1425–9. doi:10.1038/leu.2015.1.
97. Koga H, Ohshima T, Shimotohno K. Enhanced activation of tax-dependent transcription of human T-cell leukemia virus type I (HTLV-I) long terminal repeat by TORC3. J Biol Chem. 2004;279:52978–83. doi:10.1074/jbc.M409021200.
98. Koiwa T, Hamano-Usami A, Ishida T, Okayama A, Yamaguchi K, Kamihira S, Watanabe T. 5′-long terminal repeat-selective CpG methylation of latent human T-cell leukemia virus type 1 provirus in vitro and in vivo. J Virol. 2002;76:9389–97. doi:10.1128/JVI.76.18.9389-9397.2002.
99. Kondo A, Imada K, Hattori T, Yamabe H, Tanaka T, Miyasaka M, Okuma M, Uchiyama T. A model of in vivo cell proliferation of adult T-cell leukemia. Blood. 1993;82:2501–9.

100. Koralnik IJ, Fullen J, Franchini G. The p12I, p13II, and p30II proteins encoded by human T-cell leukemia/lymphotropic virus type I open reading frames I and II are localized in three different cellular compartments. J Virol. 1993;67:2360–6.
101. Koyanagi Y, Itoyama Y, Nakamura N, Takamatsu K, Kira J, Iwamasa T, Goto I, Yamamoto N. In vivo infection of human T-cell leukemia virus type I in non-T cells. Virology. 1993;196:25–33.
102. Krueger A, Fas SC, Giaisi M, Bleumink M, Merling A, Stumpf C, Baumann S, Holtkotte D, Bosch V, Krammer PH, Li-Weber M. HTLV-1 Tax protects against CD95-mediated apoptosis by induction of the cellular FLICE-inhibitory protein (c-FLIP). Blood. 2006;107:3933–9. doi:10.1182/blood-2005-06-2567.
103. Ku SCY, Lee J, Lau J, Gurumurthy M, Ng R, Lwa SH, Lee J, Klase Z, Kashanchi F, Chao S-H. XBP-1, a novel human T-lymphotropic virus type 1 (HTLV-1) tax binding protein, activates HTLV-1 basal and tax-activated transcription. J Virol. 2008;82:4343–53. doi:10.1128/JVI.02054-07.
104. Kwok RP, Laurance ME, Lundblad JR, Goldman PS, Shih H, Connor LM, Marriott SJ, Goodman RH. Control of cAMP-regulated enhancers by the viral transactivator Tax through CREB and the co-activator CBP. Nature. 1996;380:642–6. doi:10.1038/380642a0.
105. Lairmore MD, Albrecht B, D'Souza C, Nisbet JW, Ding W, Bartoe JT, Green PL, Zhang W. In vitro and in vivo functional analysis of human T cell lymphotropic virus type 1 pX open reading frames I and II. AIDS Res Hum Retrovir. 2000;16:1757–64. doi:10.1089/08892220050193272.
106. Lairmore MD, Silverman L, Ratner L. Animal models for human T-lymphotropic virus type 1 (HTLV-1) infection and transformation. Oncogene. 2005;24:6005–15. doi:10.1038/sj.onc.1208974.
107. Lambert S, Bouttier M, Vassy R, Seigneuret M, Petrow-Sadowski C, Janvier S, Heveker N, Ruscetti FW, Perret G, Jones KS, Pique C. HTLV-1 uses HSPG and neuropilin-1 for entry by molecular mimicry of VEGF165. Blood. 2009;113:5176–85. doi:10.1182/blood-2008-04-150342.
108. Lee DK, Kim B-C, Brady JN, Jeang K-T, Kim S-J. Human T-cell lymphotropic virus type 1 tax inhibits transforming growth factor-beta signaling by blocking the association of Smad proteins with Smad-binding element. J Biol Chem. 2002;277:33766–75. doi:10.1074/jbc.M200150200.
109. Lemasson I, Lewis MR, Polakowski N, Hivin P, Cavanagh M-H, Thébault S, Barbeau B, Nyborg JK, Mesnard J-M. Human T-cell leukemia virus type 1 (HTLV-1) bZIP protein interacts with the cellular transcription factor CREB to inhibit HTLV-1 transcription. J Virol. 2007;81:1543–53. doi:10.1128/JVI.00480-06.
110. Lemoine FJ, Kao SY, Marriott SJ. Suppression of DNA repair by HTLV type 1 Tax correlates with Tax trans-activation of proliferating cell nuclear antigen gene expression. AIDS Res Hum Retrovir. 2000;16:1623–7. doi:10.1089/08892220050193056.
111. Liu B, Hong S, Tang Z, Yu H, Giam C-Z. HTLV-I Tax directly binds the Cdc20-associated anaphase-promoting complex and activates it ahead of schedule. Proc Natl Acad Sci U S A. 2005;102:63–8. doi:10.1073/pnas.0406424101.
112. Low KG, Chu HM, Schwartz PM, Daniels GM, Melner MH, Comb MJ. Novel interactions between human T-cell leukemia virus type I Tax and activating transcription factor 3 at a cyclic AMP-responsive element. Mol Cell Biol. 1994;14:4958–74.
113. Ma G, Yasunaga J, Fan J, Yanagawa S, Matsuoka M. HTLV-1 bZIP factor dysregulates the Wnt pathways to support proliferation and migration of adult T-cell leukemia cells. Oncogene. 2012;32:4222–30. doi:10.1038/onc.2012.450.
114. Ma Y, Zheng S, Wang Y, Zang W, Li M, Wang N, Li P, Jin J, Dong Z, Zhao G. The HTLV-1 HBZ protein inhibits cyclin D1 expression through interacting with the cellular transcription factor CREB. Mol Biol Rep. 2013;40:5967–75. doi:10.1007/s11033-013-2706-0.
115. Macaire H, Riquet A, Moncollin V, Biémont-Trescol M-C, Duc Dodon M, Hermine O, Debaud A-L, Mahieux R, Mesnard J-M, Pierre M, Gazzolo L, Bonnefoy N, Valentin H. Tax

protein-induced expression of antiapoptotic Bfl-1 protein contributes to survival of human T-cell leukemia virus type 1 (HTLV-1)-infected T-cells. J Biol Chem. 2012;287:21357–70. doi:10.1074/jbc.M112.340992.
116. Macatonia SE, Cruickshank JK, Rudge P, Knight SC. Dendritic cells from patients with tropical spastic paraparesis are infected with HTLV-1 and stimulate autologous lymphocyte proliferation. AIDS Res Hum Retrovir. 1992;8:1699–706. doi:10.1089/aid.1992.8.1699.
117. Macnamara A, Rowan A, Hilburn S, Kadolsky U, Fujiwara H, Suemori K, Yasukawa M, Taylor G, Bangham CRM, Asquith B. HLA class I binding of HBZ determines outcome in HTLV-1 infection. PLoS Pathog. 2010;6:e1001117. doi:10.1371/journal.ppat.1001117.
118. Majone F, Jeang K-T. Unstabilized DNA breaks in HTLV-1 Tax expressing cells correlate with functional targeting of Ku80, not PKcs, XRCC4, or H2AX. Cell Biosci. 2012;2:15. doi:10.1186/2045-3701-2-15.
119. Majorovits E, Nejmeddine M, Tanaka Y, Taylor GP, Fuller SD, Bangham CRM. Human T-lymphotropic virus-1 visualized at the virological synapse by electron tomography. PLoS ONE. 2008;3:e2251. doi:10.1371/journal.pone.0002251.
120. Manel N, Kim FJ, Kinet S, Taylor N, Sitbon M, Battini J-L. The ubiquitous glucose transporter GLUT-1 is a receptor for HTLV. Cell. 2003;115:449–59.
121. Marriott SJ, Semmes OJ. Impact of HTLV-I Tax on cell cycle progression and the cellular DNA damage repair response. Oncogene. 2005;24:5986–95. doi:10.1038/sj.onc.1208976.
122. Martin-Latil S, Gnädig NF, Mallet A, Desdouits M, Guivel-Benhassine F, Jeannin P, Prévost M-C, Schwartz O, Gessain A, Ozden S, Ceccaldi P-E. Transcytosis of HTLV-1 across a tight human epithelial barrier and infection of subepithelial dendritic cells. Blood. 2012;120:572–80. doi:10.1182/blood-2011-08-374637.
123. Matsumoto J, Ohshima T, Isono O, Shimotohno K. HTLV-1 HBZ suppresses AP-1 activity by impairing both the DNA-binding ability and the stability of c-Jun protein. Oncogene. 2005;24:1001–10. doi:10.1038/sj.onc.1208297.
124. Matsuoka M, Green PL. The HBZ gene, a key player in HTLV-1 pathogenesis. Retrovirology. 2009;6:71. doi:10.1186/1742-4690-6-71.
125. Matsuoka M, Jeang KT. Human T-cell leukemia virus type 1 (HTLV-1) and leukemic transformation: viral infectivity, Tax, HBZ and therapy. Oncogene. 2011;30:1379–89. doi:10.1038/onc.2010.537.
126. Mazurov D, Ilinskaya A, Heidecker G, Lloyd P, Derse D. Quantitative comparison of HTLV-1 and HIV-1 cell-to-cell infection with new replication dependent vectors. PLoS Pathog. 2010;6:e1000788. doi:10.1371/journal.ppat.1000788.
127. Miyoshi I, Kubonishi I, Yoshimoto S, Akagi T, Ohtsuki Y, Shiraishi Y, Nagata K, Hinuma Y. Type C virus particles in a cord T-cell line derived by co-cultivating normal human cord leukocytes and human leukaemic T cells. Nature. 1981;294:770–1.
128. Mukai R, Ohshima T. HTLV-1 bZIP factor suppresses the centromere protein B (CENP-B)-mediated trimethylation of histone H3K9 through the abrogation of DNA-binding ability of CENP-B. J Gen Virol. 2014; doi:10.1099/vir.0.070201-0.
129. Nejmeddine M, Negi VS, Mukherjee S, Tanaka Y, Orth K, Taylor GP, Bangham CRM. HTLV-1-Tax and ICAM-1 act on T-cell signal pathways to polarize the microtubule-organizing center at the virological synapse. Blood. 2009;114:1016–25. doi:10.1182/blood-2008-03-136770.
130. Nicot C, Mahieux R, Takemoto S, Franchini G. Bcl-X(L) is up-regulated by HTLV-I and HTLV-II in vitro and in ex vivo ATLL samples. Blood. 2000;96:275–81.
131. Nicot C, Mulloy JC, Ferrari MG, Johnson JM, Fu K, Fukumoto R, Trovato R, Fullen J, Leonard WJ, Franchini G. HTLV-1 p12(I) protein enhances STAT5 activation and decreases the interleukin-2 requirement for proliferation of primary human peripheral blood mononuclear cells. Blood. 2001;98:823–9.
132. Ohshima T, Mukai R, Nakahara N, Matsumoto J, Isono O, Kobayashi Y, Takahashi S, Shimotohno K. HTLV-1 basic leucine-zipper factor, HBZ, interacts with MafB and

suppresses transcription through a Maf recognition element. J Cell Biochem. 2010;111:187–94. doi:10.1002/jcb.22687.
133. Ohsugi T. A transgenic mouse model of human T cell leukemia virus type 1-associated diseases. Front Microbiol. 2013;4:49. doi:10.3389/fmicb.2013.00049.
134. Ohtani K, Iwanaga R, Arai M, Huang Y, Matsumura Y, Nakamura M. Cell type-specific E2F activation and cell cycle progression induced by the oncogene product Tax of human T-cell leukemia virus type I. J Biol Chem. 2000;275:11154–63.
135. Okamoto K, Fujisawa J-I, Reth M, Yonehara S. Human T-cell leukemia virus type-I oncoprotein Tax inhibits Fas-mediated apoptosis by inducing cellular FLIP through activation of NF-kappaB. Genes Cells. 2006;11:177–91. doi:10.1111/j.1365-2443.2006.00927.x.
136. Ooms M, Krikoni A, Kress AK, Simon V, Münk C. APOBEC3A, APOBEC3B, and APOBEC3H haplotype 2 restrict human T-lymphotropic virus type 1. J Virol. 2012;86:6097–108. doi:10.1128/JVI.06570-11.
137. Pais-Correia A-M, Sachse M, Guadagnini S, Robbiati V, Lasserre R, Gessain A, Gout O, Alcover A, Thoulouze M-I. Biofilm-like extracellular viral assemblies mediate HTLV-1 cell-to-cell transmission at virological synapses. Nat Med. 2010;16:83–9. doi:10.1038/nm.2065.
138. Park HU, Jeong J-H, Chung JH, Brady JN. Human T-cell leukemia virus type 1 Tax interacts with Chk1 and attenuates DNA-damage induced G2 arrest mediated by Chk1. Oncogene. 2004;23:4966–74. doi:10.1038/sj.onc.1207644.
139. Park HU, Jeong S-J, Jeong J-H, Chung JH, Brady JN. Human T-cell leukemia virus type 1 Tax attenuates gamma-irradiation-induced apoptosis through physical interaction with Chk2. Oncogene. 2006;25:438–47. doi:10.1038/sj.onc.1209059.
140. Peloponese J-M, Jeang K-T. Role for Akt/protein kinase B and activator protein-1 in cellular proliferation induced by the human T-cell leukemia virus type 1 tax oncoprotein. J Biol Chem. 2006;281:8927–38. doi:10.1074/jbc.M510598200.
141. Philip S, Zahoor MA, Zhi H, Ho Y-K, Giam C-Z. Regulation of human T-lymphotropic virus type I latency and reactivation by HBZ and Rex. PLoS Pathog. 2014;10:e1004040. doi:10.1371/journal.ppat.1004040.
142. Philpott SM, Buehring GC. Defective DNA repair in cells with human T-cell leukemia/bovine leukemia viruses: role of tax gene. J Natl Cancer Inst. 1999;91:933–42.
143. Pique C, Jones KS. Pathways of cell-cell transmission of HTLV-1. Front Microbiol. 2012;3:378. doi:10.3389/fmicb.2012.00378.
144. Pise-Masison CA, Mahieux R, Jiang H, Ashcroft M, Radonovich M, Duvall J, Guillerm C, Brady JN. Inactivation of p53 by human T-cell lymphotropic virus type 1 Tax requires activation of the NF-kappaB pathway and is dependent on p53 phosphorylation. Mol Cell Biol. 2000;20:3377–86.
145. Poiesz BJ, Ruscetti FW, Gazdar AF, Bunn PA, Minna JD, Gallo RC. Detection and isolation of type C retrovirus particles from fresh and cultured lymphocytes of a patient with cutaneous T-cell lymphoma. Proc Natl Acad Sci U S A. 1980;77:7415–9.
146. Reddy TR, Tang H, Li X, Wong-Staal F. Functional interaction of the HTLV-1 transactivator Tax with activating transcription factor-4 (ATF4). Oncogene. 1997;14:2785–92. doi:10.1038/sj.onc.1201119.
147. Reid RL, Lindholm PF, Mireskandari A, Dittmer J, Brady JN. Stabilization of wild-type p53 in human T-lymphocytes transformed by HTLV-I. Oncogene. 1993;8:3029–36.
148. Robek MD, Ratner L. Immortalization of CD4(+) and CD8(+) T lymphocytes by human T-cell leukemia virus type 1 Tax mutants expressed in a functional molecular clone. J Virol. 1999;73:4856–65.
149. Robek MD, Wong FH, Ratner L. Human T-cell leukemia virus type 1 pX-I and pX-II open reading frames are dispensable for the immortalization of primary lymphocytes. J Virol. 1998;72:4458–62.
150. Rous P. A sarcoma of the fowl transmissible by an agent separable from the tumor cells. J Exp Med. 1911;13:397–411.

151. Santiago F, Clark E, Chong S, Molina C, Mozafari F, Mahieux R, Fujii M, Azimi N, Kashanchi F. Transcriptional up-regulation of the cyclin D2 gene and acquisition of new cyclin-dependent kinase partners in human T-cell leukemia virus type 1-infected cells. J Virol. 1999;73:9917–27.
152. Satou Y, Yasunaga J-I, Yoshida M, Matsuoka M. HTLV-I basic leucine zipper factor gene mRNA supports proliferation of adult T cell leukemia cells. Proc Natl Acad Sci U S A. 2006;103:720–5. doi:10.1073/pnas.0507631103.
153. Satou Y, Yasunaga J-I, Zhao T, Yoshida M, Miyazato P, Takai K, Shimizu K, Ohshima K, Green PL, Ohkura N, Yamaguchi T, Ono M, Sakaguchi S, Matsuoka M. HTLV-1 bZIP factor induces T-cell lymphoma and systemic inflammation in vivo. PLoS Pathog. 2011;7: e1001274. doi:10.1371/journal.ppat.1001274.
154. Seiki M, Hattori S, Hirayama Y, Yoshida M. Human adult T-cell leukemia virus: complete nucleotide sequence of the provirus genome integrated in leukemia cell DNA. Proc Natl Acad Sci U S A. 1983;80:3618–22.
155. Seiki M, Hikikoshi A, Taniguchi T, Yoshida M. Expression of the pX gene of HTLV-I: general splicing mechanism in the HTLV family. Science. 1985;228:1532–4.
156. Silic-Benussi M, Cannizzaro E, Venerando A, Cavallari I, Petronilli V, La Rocca N, Marin O, Chieco-Bianchi L, Di Lisa F, D'Agostino DM, Bernardi P, Ciminale V. Modulation of mitochondrial K(+) permeability and reactive oxygen species production by the p13 protein of human T-cell leukemia virus type 1. Biochim Biophys Acta. 2009;1787:947–54. doi:10.1016/j.bbabio.2009.02.001.
157. Silic-Benussi M, Cavallari I, Zorzan T, Rossi E, Hiraragi H, Rosato A, Horie K, Saggioro D, Lairmore MD, Willems L, Chieco-Bianchi L, D'Agostino DM, Ciminale V. Suppression of tumor growth and cell proliferation by p13II, a mitochondrial protein of human T cell leukemia virus type 1. Proc Natl Acad Sci U S A. 2004;101:6629–34. doi:10.1073/pnas.0305502101.
158. Siu Y-T, Chin K-T, Siu K-L, Yee Wai Choy E, Jeang K-T, Jin D-Y. TORC1 and TORC2 coactivators are required for tax activation of the human T-cell leukemia virus type 1 long terminal repeats. J Virol. 2006;80:7052–9. doi:10.1128/JVI.00103-06.
159. Sodroski JG, Rosen CA, Haseltine WA. Trans-acting transcriptional activation of the long terminal repeat of human T lymphotropic viruses in infected cells. Science. 1984;225:381–5.
160. Sugata K, Satou Y, Yasunaga J-I, Hara H, Ohshima K, Utsunomiya A, Mitsuyama M, Matsuoka M. HTLV-1 bZIP factor impairs cell-mediated immunity by suppressing production of Th1 cytokines. Blood. 2012;119:434–44. doi:10.1182/blood-2011-05-357459.
161. Sun S-C, Yamaoka S. Activation of NF-kappaB by HTLV-I and implications for cell transformation. Oncogene. 2005;24:5952–64. doi:10.1038/sj.onc.1208969.
162. Suzuki T, Hirai H, Fujisawa J, Fujita T, Yoshida M. A trans-activator Tax of human T-cell leukemia virus type 1 binds to NF-kappa B p50 and serum response factor (SRF) and associates with enhancer DNAs of the NF-kappa B site and CArG box. Oncogene. 1993;8:2391–7.
163. Swaims AY, Khani F, Zhang Y, Roberts AI, Devadas S, Shi Y, Rabson AB. Immune activation induces immortalization of HTLV-1 LTR-Tax transgenic CD4+ T cells. Blood. 2010;116:2994–3003. doi:10.1182/blood-2009-07-231050.
164. Sze A, Belgnaoui SM, Olagnier D, Lin R, Hiscott J, van Grevenynghe J. Host restriction factor SAMHD1 limits human T cell leukemia virus type 1 infection of monocytes via STING-mediated apoptosis. Cell Host Microbe. 2013;14:422–34. doi:10.1016/j.chom.2013.09.009.
165. Tabakin-Fix Y, Azran I, Schavinky-Khrapunsky Y, Levy O, Aboud M. Functional inactivation of p53 by human T-cell leukemia virus type 1 Tax protein: mechanisms and clinical implications. Carcinogenesis. 2006;27:673–81. doi:10.1093/carcin/bgi274.
166. Takachi T, Takahashi M, Takahashi-Yoshita M, Higuchi M, Obata M, Mishima Y, Okuda S, Tanaka Y, Matsuoka M, Saitoh A, Green PL, Fujii M. Human T-cell leukemia virus type

1 Tax oncoprotein represses the expression of the BCL11B tumor suppressor in T-cells. Cancer Sci. 2015;106:461–5. doi:10.1111/cas.12618.
167. Takeda S, Maeda M, Morikawa S, Taniguchi Y, Yasunaga J-I, Nosaka K, Tanaka Y, Matsuoka M. Genetic and epigenetic inactivation of tax gene in adult T-cell leukemia cells. Int J Cancer. 2004;109:559–67. doi:10.1002/ijc.20007.
168. Takeuchi H, Takahashi M, Norose Y, Takeshita T, Fukunaga Y, Takahashi H. Transformation of breast milk macrophages by HTLV-I: implications for HTLV-I transmission via breastfeeding. Biomed Res. 2010;31:53–61.
169. Tanaka-Nakanishi A, Yasunaga J-I, Takai K, Matsuoka M. HTLV-1 bZIP factor suppresses apoptosis by attenuating the function of FoxO3a and altering its localization. Cancer Res. 2014;74:188–200. doi:10.1158/0008-5472.CAN-13-0436.
170. Taylor JM, Ghorbel S, Nicot C. Genome wide analysis of human genes transcriptionally and post-transcriptionally regulated by the HTLV-I protein p30. BMC Genomics. 2009;10:311. doi:10.1186/1471-2164-10-311.
171. Tezuka K, Xun R, Tei M, Ueno T, Tanaka M, Takenouchi N, Fujisawa J-I. An animal model of adult T-cell leukemia: humanized mice with HTLV-1-specific immunity. Blood. 2014;123:346–55. doi:10.1182/blood-2013-06-508861.
172. Thébault S, Basbous J, Hivin P, Devaux C, Mesnard J-M. HBZ interacts with JunD and stimulates its transcriptional activity. FEBS Lett. 2004;562:165–70. doi:10.1016/S0014-5793(04)00225-X.
173. Tochikura T, Iwahashi M, Matsumoto T, Koyanagi Y, Hinuma Y, Yamamoto N. Effect of human serum anti-HTLV antibodies on viral antigen induction in vitro cultured peripheral lymphocytes from adult T-cell leukemia patients and healthy virus carriers. Int J Cancer. 1985;36:1–7.
174. Toyoshima H, Itoh M, Inoue J, Seiki M, Takaku F, Yoshida M. Secondary structure of the human T-cell leukemia virus type 1 rex-responsive element is essential for rex regulation of RNA processing and transport of unspliced RNAs. J Virol. 1990;64:2825–32.
175. Tsujimoto A, Nyunoya H, Morita T, Sato T, Shimotohno K. Isolation of cDNAs for DNA-binding proteins which specifically bind to a tax-responsive enhancer element in the long terminal repeat of human T-cell leukemia virus type I. J Virol. 1991;65:1420–6.
176. Tsukahara T, Kannagi M, Ohashi T, Kato H, Arai M, Nunez G, Iwanaga Y, Yamamoto N, Ohtani K, Nakamura M, Fujii M. Induction of Bcl-x(L) expression by human T-cell leukemia virus type 1 Tax through NF-kappaB in apoptosis-resistant T-cell transfectants with Tax. J Virol. 1999;73:7981–7.
177. Tugizov SM, Herrera R, Veluppillai P, Greenspan D, Soros V, Greene WC, Levy JA, Palefsky JM. Differential transmission of HIV traversing fetal oral/intestinal epithelia and adult oral epithelia. J Virol. 2012;86:2556–70. doi:10.1128/JVI.06578-11.
178. Uchiyama T, Yodoi J, Sagawa K, Takatsuki K, Uchino H. Adult T-cell leukemia: clinical and hematologic features of 16 cases. Blood. 1977;50:481–92.
179. Unge T, Solomin L, Mellini M, Derse D, Felber BK, Pavlakis GN. The Rex regulatory protein of human T-cell lymphotropic virus type I binds specifically to its target site within the viral RNA. Proc Natl Acad Sci U S A. 1991;88:7145–9.
180. Usui T, Yanagihara K, Tsukasaki K, Murata K, Hasegawa H, Yamada Y, Kamihira S. Characteristic expression of HTLV-1 basic zipper factor (HBZ) transcripts in HTLV-1 provirus-positive cells. Retrovirology. 2008;5:34. doi:10.1186/1742-4690-5-34.
181. Valeri VW, Hryniewicz A, Andresen V, Jones K, Fenizia C, Bialuk I, Chung H-K, Fukumoto R, Parks RW, Ferrari MG, Nicot C, Cecchinato V, Ruscetti F, Franchini G. Requirement of the human T-cell leukemia virus p12 and p30 products for infectivity of human dendritic cells and macaques but not rabbits. Blood. 2010;116:3809–17. doi:10.1182/blood-2010-05-284141.
182. Van Prooyen N, Gold H, Andresen V, Schwartz O, Jones K, Ruscetti F, Lockett S, Gudla P, Venzon D, Franchini G. Human T-cell leukemia virus type 1 p8 protein increases cellular

conduits and virus transmission. Proc Natl Acad Sci. 2010;107:20738–43. doi:10.1073/pnas.1009635107.
183. Vernin C, Thenoz M, Pinatel C, Gessain A, Gout O, Delfau-Larue M-H, Nazaret N, Legras-Lachuer C, Wattel E, Mortreux F. HTLV-1 bZIP factor HBZ promotes cell proliferation and genetic instability by activating OncomiRs. Cancer Res. 2014;74:6082–93. doi:10.1158/0008-5472.CAN-13-3564.
184. Villaudy J, Wencker M, Gadot N, Gillet NA, Scoazec J-Y, Gazzolo L, Manz MG, Bangham CRM, Dodon MD. HTLV-1 propels thymic human T cell development in "human immune system" Rag2$^{-}$/$^{-}$ gamma c$^{-}$/$^{-}$ mice. PLoS Pathog. 2011;7:e1002231–1. doi:10.1371/journal.ppat.1002231.
185. Watanabe S, Ohta S, Yajima M, Terashima K, Ito M, Mugishima H, Fujiwara S, Shimizu K, Honda M, Shimizu N, Yamamoto N. Humanized NOD/SCID/IL2Rgamma(null) mice transplanted with hematopoietic stem cells under nonmyeloablative conditions show prolonged life spans and allow detailed analysis of human immunodeficiency virus type 1 pathogenesis. J Virol. 2007;81:13259–64. doi:10.1128/JVI.01353-07.
186. Watanabe T, Seiki M, Yoshida M. Retrovirus terminology. Science. 1983;222:1178.
187. Xiao G, Fu J. NF-κB and cancer: a paradigm of Yin-Yang. Am J Cancer Res. 2011;1:192–221.
188. Yajima M, Imadome K-I, Nakagawa A, Watanabe S, Terashima K, Nakamura H, Ito M, Shimizu N, Honda M, Yamamoto N, Fujiwara S. A new humanized mouse model of Epstein-Barr virus infection that reproduces persistent infection, lymphoproliferative disorder, and cell-mediated and humoral immune responses. J Infect Dis. 2008;198:673–82. doi:10.1086/590502.
189. Yamagishi M, Katano H, Hishima T, Shimoyama T, Ota Y, Nakano K, Ishida T, Okada S, Watanabe T. Coordinated loss of microRNA group causes defenseless signaling in malignant lymphoma. Sci Rep. 2015;5:17868. doi:10.1038/srep17868.
190. Yasunaga J, Jeang K-T. Viral transformation and aneuploidy. Environ Mol Mutagen. 2009;50:733–40. doi:10.1002/em.20480.
191. Ye J, Silverman L, Lairmore MD, Green PL. HTLV-1 Rex is required for viral spread and persistence in vivo but is dispensable for cellular immortalization in vitro. Blood. 2003;102:3963–9. doi:10.1182/blood-2003-05-1490.
192. Yeung ML, Yasunaga J-I, Bennasser Y, Dusetti N, Harris D, Ahmad N, Matsuoka M, Jeang K-T. Roles for microRNAs, miR-93 and miR-130b, and tumor protein 53-induced nuclear protein 1 tumor suppressor in cell growth dysregulation by human T-cell lymphotropic virus 1. Cancer Res. 2008;68:8976–85. doi:10.1158/0008-5472.CAN-08-0769.
193. Yoshida M, Miyoshi I, Hinuma Y. Isolation and characterization of retrovirus from cell lines of human adult T-cell leukemia and its implication in the disease. Proc Natl Acad Sci U S A. 1982;79:2031–5.
194. Yoshimura T, Fujisawa J, Yoshida M. Multiple cDNA clones encoding nuclear proteins that bind to the tax-dependent enhancer of HTLV-1: all contain a leucine zipper structure and basic amino acid domain. EMBO J. 1990;9:2537–42.
195. Zacharopoulos VR, Perotti ME, Phillips DM. Lymphocyte-facilitated infection of epithelia by human T-cell lymphotropic virus type I. J Virol. 1992;66:4601–5.
196. Zane L, Yasunaga J, Mitagami Y, Yedavalli V, Tang S-W, Chen C-Y, Ratner L, Lu X, Jeang K-T. Wip1 and p53 contribute to HTLV-1 Tax-induced tumorigenesis. Retrovirology. 2012;9:114. doi:10.1006/meth.2001.1262.
197. Zhao LJ, Giam CZ. Human T-cell lymphotropic virus type I (HTLV-I) transcriptional activator, Tax, enhances CREB binding to HTLV-I 21-base-pair repeats by protein-protein interaction. Proc Natl Acad Sci U S A. 1992;89:7070–4.
198. Zhao T, Satou Y, Sugata K, Miyazato P, Green PL, Imamura T, Matsuoka M. HTLV-1 bZIP factor enhances TGF-β signaling through p300 coactivator. Blood. 2011;118:1865–76. doi:10.1182/blood-2010-12-326199.

199. Zhao T, Yasunaga J-I, Satou Y, Nakao M, Takahashi M, Fujii M, Matsuoka M. Human T-cell leukemia virus type 1 bZIP factor selectively suppresses the classical pathway of NF-kappaB. Blood. 2009;113:2755–64. doi:10.1182/blood-2008-06-161729.
200. Zhi H, Yang L, Kuo Y-L, Ho Y-K, Shih H-M, Giam C-Z. NF-κB hyper-activation by HTLV-1 tax induces cellular senescence, but can be alleviated by the viral anti-sense protein HBZ. PLoS Pathog. 2011;7:e1002025. doi:10.1371/journal.ppat.1002025.

# Chapter 3
# Epidemiology

**Masako Iwanaga**

## 3.1 Introduction

Adult T-cell leukemia-lymphoma (ATL) is a malignancy of peripheral T lymphocytes caused by human T-cell leukemia virus type 1 (HTLV-1). In 1977, ATL was first reported as a distinct clinical entity in Japan [79, 89], and HTLV-1 was subsequently discovered as the causative agent of ATL [59, 98]. The first set of diagnostic criteria for ATL and the four clinical subtypes (acute, lymphoma, chronic, and smoldering) were proposed based on the prognostic factors, clinical features, and the natural history of the disease in 1991 [71]. The causal etiological association of HTLV-1 with ATL was established on the basis of a broad range of experimental and epidemiological evidence in the early 1980s, including that all ATL patients have antibodies against HTLV-1 [24, 25], geographical areas of high incidence of ATL patients correspond closely with areas of high incidence of HTLV-1 carriers [81], HTLV-1 immortalizes human CD4 T cells in vitro [21], and monoclonal integration of HTLV-1 provirus DNA was demonstrated in ATL cells [95]. Nevertheless, the current molecular, clinical, and epidemiological evidence is insufficient to understand fully what determines who will and who will not develop ATL among HTLV-1 carriers. This chapter reviews available information on the epidemiological aspects of HTLV-1 and ATL and the risk factors for the development of ATL from HTLV-1 carriers.

M. Iwanaga (✉)
Department of Frontier Life Science, Nagasaki University Graduate School of Biomedical Sciences, Sakamoto 1-12-4, Nagasaki 852-8523, Japan
e-mail: masakoiwng@nagasaki-u.ac.jp



T. Watanabe, T. Fukushima (eds.), *Adult T-cell Leukemia/Lymphoma*,
DOI 10.1007/978-4-431-56523-9_3

## 3.2 Prevalence, Incidence, and Lifetime Risk

### *3.2.1 Prevalence and Geographic Distribution of HTLV-1*

The exact numbers of HTLV-1-seropositive individuals and ATL patients worldwide are unknown. Several studies have estimated the worldwide prevalence of HTLV-1, but few for ATL. Areas with HTLV-1 seroprevalence >1% are recognized as highly endemic regions [17]. Given that ATL occurs exclusively in areas endemic for HTLV-1 [29], it is useful to know the geographic distribution of HTLV-1 infection.

From the late 1980s to 1990s, HTLV-1 seroscreening was vigorously conducted worldwide. Currently, Southwestern Japan, sub-Saharan Africa, South America, the Caribbean islands, and part of the Middle East and Australo-Melanesia are recognized as the major endemic regions for HTLV-1 (summarized by Proietti et al. [62]). The number of HTLV-1 carriers worldwide was estimated to be ~20 million in 1993 [13] and ~10 million in 2012 [18].

In Asia, Japan is one of the most endemic regions for HTLV-1. Within Japan, there is uneven distribution of endemic foci, such as southwestern districts (Kyushu and Okinawa), coastal areas of Shikoku and Kinki, and other microendemic regions. The overall HTLV-1 seroprevalence in blood donors was reported to be 1–6% in the 1980s [78] and 0.1–2% in 2006 [66]. The number of HTLV-1-infected individuals in Japan was estimated to be around one million in 1990 [78] and 2012 [66]. In other Asian regions, a low HTLV-1 seroprevalence was reported in China (0.013–0.06%), Korea (0.007–0.25%), Taiwan (0.058–0.82%), India (0.14%), and Israel (0.001%), in all of which only a few cases of ATL were reported [18].

In Middle East, Mashhad, a northeastern part of Iran, is a known endemic area for HTLV-1 with a seroprevalence of 0.7–3% [1, 63].

In Oceania, a high HTLV-1 seroprevalence and non-negligible number of patients with ATL and HTLV-1-associated myelopathy/tropical spastic paraparesis (HAM/TSP) have been reported among Aboriginal populations in Central Australia [14], Papua New Guinea, and the Solomon Islands [18]. Interestingly, HTLV-1 strain subtype in Oceania is distinct from those in other regions. Among seven HTLV-1 strain subtypes (a–g), the Cosmopolitan subtype (a) has spread worldwide, and the African subtypes (b and d–g) have spread in African and Caribbean regions, but the Australo-Melanesian subtype (c) is found only in Oceania [92].

In the USA, HTLV-1 prevalence has been studied extensively in blood donors. The Retrovirus Epidemiology Donor Study Group reported that the HTLV-1 seroprevalence among first-time blood donors was 0.009% during 1991–1995 [70] and 0.0051% during 2000–2009 [11]. Most of the HTLV-1-positive individuals were Asians from Japan or Blacks from the Caribbean regions.

The Caribbean regions (including Jamaica, Haiti, and Martinique) and Brazil are the most endemic regions for HTLV-1 infection [18]. The majority of HTLV-1-infected people are of African ancestry from areas endemic for HTLV-1 and ATL. HTLV-1 prevalence in the Caribbean regions is up to 17.4% [49]. In Brazil, HTLV-1 prevalence among first-time blood donors was 0.14% during 2007–2009, and the prevalence differed by region, from 0.08% to 0.22% [9]. In particular, Salvador da Bahia, located on the northeast coast of Brazil, is the highest endemic area for HTLV-1.

In Africa, HTLV-1 seroprevalence among the general population varies from low in North Africa (e.g., Morocco, 0.6%) to high in sub-Saharan countries (Cameroon and Guinea-Bissau, 5%) [18]. HTLV-1 seroprevalence among pregnant women also varies from 0.7 to 5.5% [18].

In Europe, Romania is the country with the highest HTLV-1 prevalence (0.64%) among blood donors [58]. In other European countries, HTLV-1 seroprevalence in first-time blood donors is <0.004%, and patients with ATL are rare [43]. HTLV-1 carriers and ATL are also reported in France and the UK where the majority of infected people are immigrants and their descendants from a high-endemic area of HTLV-1 such as Africa and the Caribbean. In the UK, the overall HTLV-1 prevalence among pregnant women was 31 per 100,000 [2]. In France, it is estimated that there are 10,000–25,000 HTLV-1-infected persons [18].

### 3.2.2 *Incidence of ATL in the General Population*

Few population-based prospective cohort studies have investigated the risk of developing ATL. Most of the epidemiological studies of ATL have been conducted cross-sectionally through countrywide surveys or cancer registry systems (summarized in Iwanaga et al. [34]). In regional cancer registry systems, ATL patients are registered according to the International Classification of Diseases for Oncology, 3rd edition (ICD-O-3) histological code, 9827 [15]. However, information on clinical subtype of ATL is not available in regional cancer registry systems because there is no ICD-O-3 code for the subtypes.

In Japan, ATL accounts for 40–50% of non-Hodgkin lymphoma (NHL) in HTLV-1-endemic areas [4, 55], but for only 10% of NHL throughout Japan [3]. A series of nationwide hospital-based surveys reported 700–800 new cases of ATL annually during 1986–1997 [82] and 910 cases in 2006–2007 [94]. Based on these surveys, the estimated number of annual new cases of ATL in Japan was ~1,000 cases. The mean age at diagnosis of ATL has increased with time, from the early 50s in 1980–1990 to the late 60s in 2006–2007. Regarding subtype distribution, lymphoma subtype tended to increase with time from 19.1% of all ATL in 1984–1987 [71], to 23.7% in 1980–1990 [82], and 34.8% in 2006–2007 [94] (Fig. 3.1). A recent analysis of 15 population-based cancer registries in Japan estimated annual age-standardized incidence of ATL during 1993–2006 was 2.53–2.09 (per 100,000 persons, standardized to the world population) for men and 1.66–1.67 for women in endemic regions, whereas 0.10–0.21 for men and 0.09–0.14 for women in nonendemic regions [12]. They also reported that the annual incidence was declining in endemic regions but increasing in nonendemic regions. Unfortunately,

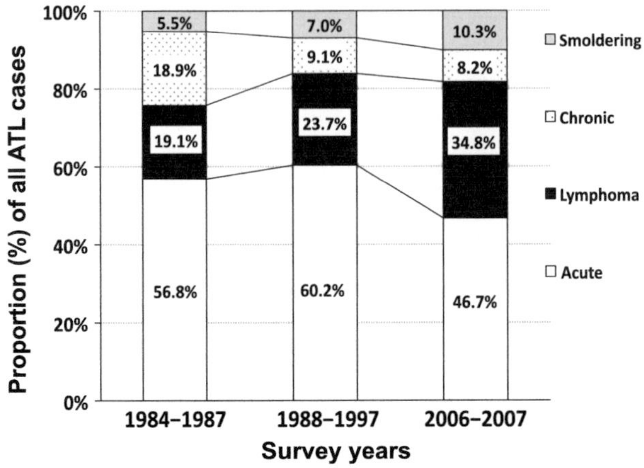


**Fig. 3.1** Changes in proportion of ATL subtype (acute, lymphoma, chronic, and smoldering types) over time. The percentage shows the proportion of each subtype in the total number of ATL cases in the respective survey duration (The data for 1984–1987 and 1988–1997 were taken from reports of the Lymphoma Study Group in Japan [71, 82], and the data for 2006–2007 were based on a report by Yamada et al. [94])

insufficient data for ATL have been accumulated in regional cancer registries in Japan.

In the USA, most patients with ATL are migrants from endemic areas. A population-based survey reported that the annual incidence of ATL in African Americans in Brooklyn was estimated to be 3.2 per 100,000 person-years [44]. The North American Association of Central Cancer Registries [96] reported a total of 431 cases (248 men and 183 women) of ATL between 1997 and 2002, showing that the age-adjusted incidence rate was 0.05 for men and 0.03 for women per 100,000 population. The study also reported a racial difference in the incidence, showing that African Americans had the highest rates of ATL (0.12 for men and 0.13 for women per 100,000 population). This observation can be explained by the higher number of migrants from endemic areas of the Caribbean and parts of sub-Saharan Africa rather than a racial difference in susceptibility.

In Brazil, ATL accounts for ~30% of patients with T-cell malignancies [61]. A Brazilian ATL Study Group identified 195 cases of ATL in the national registry of T-cell malignancies in 1994–1998 [60], but no epidemiological indicators were available.

### *3.2.3 Incidence and Lifetime Risk of ATL Among HTLV-1 Carriers*

Few prospective studies have investigated development of ATL among asymptomatic HTLV-1 carriers. Most studies have evaluated cross-sectionally the incidence of ATL by a linkage between age- and sex-specific ATL incidence in regional cancer registries and age- and sex-specific seroprevalence data of blood donors or hospital patients.

*In Japan*, crude annual incidence of ATL was reported as ~60 per 100,000 HTLV-1 carriers aged $\geq$20 years in a nationwide survey [78]: 116 for men and 66 for women per 100,000 HTLV-1 carriers in Saga (Southwest Japan) [84]; 137.7 for men and 57.4 for women per 100,000 HTLV-1 carriers aged >30 years in small islands with high HTLV-1 seroprevalence [4]; and 61 per 100,000 HTLV-1 carriers in a hospital-based study in Nagasaki (Southwest Japan) [42]. Based on these data, the cumulative lifetime risk for development of ATL in HTLV-1 carriers is estimated to be 3–5% (4–7% for men, 2–4% for women) in Japan. A recent analysis reported an annual ATL incidence among 10,000 HTLV-1 carriers of 7.7 and 8.7 for the endemic and nonendemic areas, respectively, by multiplying the seroprevalence of first-time blood donors in 2006–2007 by the number of ATL cases accumulated by a nationwide survey in 2007–2008 [65].

*In Jamaica*, Murphy et al. reported that the cumulative lifetime risk of ATL for HTLV-1 carriers before age 20 years is estimated to be 4% for men and 4.2% for women [50].

## 3.3 Risk Factors for ATL Development from HTLV-1 Carriers

HTLV-1 infection alone is not sufficient for development of ATL. A variety of host susceptibility, laboratory, viral, and immune markers, genetic abnormalities, and other factors are potential factors for the development of ATL (Table 3.1). However, so far, there is no critical determinant for progression from HTLV-1 carrier status to overt ATL.

### *3.3.1 Host Susceptibility*

There is consistent evidence that aging is a definite risk factor for the development of ATL from HTLV-1 carrier status. In Japan, ATL occurs mostly in adults and most patients with ATL are diagnosed at age >60 years [94]. In the most recent nationwide survey of ATL diagnosed during 2010–2011, 65% of patients with ATL were aged $\geq$60 years (unpublished data). In Japan, most transmission of HTLV-1 occurs during infancy through mother-to-child transmission via breastfeeding; therefore, the latent period from primary infection until ATL onset may be >60 years. In Jamaica and Brazil, however, the average age at diagnosis of ATL was reported to be 43 years and 44 years, respectively [20, 60]; thus, age at onset of ATL in the Caribbean is younger than in Japan. The reason for the difference in age at onset between Japanese and Caribbean patients is unknown. Differences in race,

**Table 3.1** Risk markers for the development of ATL in HTLV-1 carriers

| | |
|---|---|
| *Host susceptibility* | |
| | Attained at an age of >50 years |
| | Male sex |
| | Mother-to-child infection in infancy |
| | HLA-A26, HLA-B4002, HLA-B4006, and HLA-B4801 |
| *Immune system abnormalities* | |
| | Co-infection with *Strongyloides stercoralis* |
| | Undergoing immunosuppressive treatment |
| *Viral markers* | |
| | High HTLV-1 proviral load >4 copies/100 PBMCs |
| | Monoclonal integration of proviral DNA |
| *Laboratory markers* | |
| | High level of sIL-2R >500 U/mL |
| | High level of anti-HTLV-1 titer >1024 |
| | High level of circulating abnormal lymphocytes >0.6% |
| | High level of white blood cell count >9000/μL |
| | Low level of of anti-Tax reactivity |
| | Decreasing cell surface antigen CD26 CADM1 + CD7 |
| | Decreasing cell surface antigen ratio of CD26/CD25 |

References are described in Sect. 3.3 "Risk factor for ATL development from HTLV-1 carriers" in this chapter

*ATL* adult T-cell leukemia, *HTLV-1* human T-cell leukemia virus type 1, *HLA* human leukocyte antigen, *PBMC* peripheral blood mononuclear cell, *sIL-2R* soluble interleukin-2 receptor, *CD* cluster of differentiation

lifestyle and HTLV-1 genotype [Cosmopolitan subtype (a) in Japan vs African subtypes (b and d–g) in the Caribbean] [92], and other unknown differences may be involved.

There is consistent evidence that male sex is a definite risk factor for the development of ATL from HTLV-1 carrier status in Japan. Several Japanese cohort studies reported that male HTLV-1 carriers had a three- to fivefold higher risk of developing ATL than female carriers had [4, 27]. However, the male-to-female ratio of ATL patients with HTLV-1 African subtypes differs from the ratio in patients with Japanese subtypes: a population-based survey in Brooklyn, New York, reported that the annual incidence of ATL was three times higher in women than in men [44]. A Jamaican study also showed that the cumulative lifetime risk of ATL was higher in women (4.2%) than in men (4.0%) [50]. The reason for the sex-related differences in the incidence rate of ATL between Japan and other regions is unknown. This also may be related to the difference in HTLV-1 subtype.

Specific human leukocyte antigens (HLAs) are associated with an increased risk of developing ATL in Japan [90]. The allele frequencies of HLA-A26, HLA-B4002, HLA-B 4006, and HLA-B4801 were higher in ATL patients than in asymptomatic HTLV-1 carriers, and ATL patients possessing these alleles developed ATL 12.6 years earlier than patients with other alleles [97]. The impact of HLA alleles on the development of HTLV-1-related diseases has been investigated to explain familial clustering and ethnic differences of ATL [73, 86].

Apparent ethnic or racial differences in susceptibility to HTLV-1 infection and developing ATL seem unlikely. Studies from the USA and UK show a higher incidence of ATL in Blacks than in Whites [72, 73, 96]; however, most of the ATL patients were of African origin, particularly from areas where HTLV-1 is endemic.

### 3.3.2 *Immune System Abnormalities*

HTLV-1 infects CD4-positive T cells, and chronic infection can lead to abnormal immunity in HTLV-1 carriers. A variety of abnormalities of immunoregulatory genes has been investigated to explain the development of ATL (summarized in Matuoka et al. 2011 [46]). All of these abnormalities suggest that a higher proliferation of HTLV-1-infected cells and a low immune response against Tax may be associated with the onset of ATL.

There are many clinical reports to suggest that persistent immune abnormality contributes to the development of ATL from HTLV-1 carrier status. For example, HTLV-1 carriers co-infected with *Strongyloides stercoralis* (as an opportunistic pathogen) are considered a high-risk group for developing ATL, with a high provirus load [16, 51], high level of soluble interleukin-2 receptor (IL-2R) [69], and high level of soluble CD30 [7]. Furthermore, a lot of clinical evidence has accumulated recently to indicate the potential contribution of immunosuppression in HTLV-1 carriers to the development of ATL. For example, ATL developed from HTLV-1 carriers undergoing immunosuppressive treatment after organ transplantation [28, 39, 86, 97] and from HTLV-1 carriers with comorbid rheumatoid arthritis treated with tocilizumab or other first biological agents [8, 52]. Further studies are needed to confirm the definite association between the immunosuppressive state and the development of ATL from HTLV-1 carriers.

### 3.3.3 *Laboratory Markers*

A variety of laboratory prognostic indicators for the development of ATL from HTLV-1 carrier status have been reported. These include a high number of circulating abnormal lymphocytes, high level of soluble IL-2R (>500 U/mL), high level of lactate dehydrogenase, low anti-Tax reactivity, high HTLV-1 antibody titers, and high white blood cell count (>9000/μL), after adjustment for age, sex, and relative lymphocyte counts [26, 31, 35].

Aberrant expression of cell surface antigens is usually used for clinical routine diagnosis of ATL based on the fact that ATL cells phenotypically express CD4, CCR4, and CD25. Two studies reported that expression of CD3, CD7, and CD26 on

HTLV-1-infected cells was diminished in acute and chronic ATL and slightly downregulated in smoldering ATL [82, 86]. These results suggest that the downregulation of those cell surface antigens could be predictive markers for the early phase of leukemogenesis of ATL from HTLV-1 carriers. Kamihira et al. [36] analyzed cell surface antigens on HTLV-1-infected cells in HTLV-1 carriers, smoldering ATL, and chronic ATL, by taking into consideration the pattern of Southern blot hybridization and provirus load. The results suggest that reduced expression of CD26 and decreasing CD26/CD25 ratio are novel biomarkers for predicting clonal bands and discrimination of carriers and smoldering ATL. Kobayashi et al. [41] reported that flow cytometry of T cells revealed that expression of cell adhesion molecule 1 (CADM1) and stepwise downregulation of CD7 were closely associated with the clonal expansion of HTLV-1-infected cells in ATL. They also showed that CADM1$^{+}$ cells with downregulated expression of CD7 in asymptomatic HTLV-1 carriers exhibited properties in common with those in indolent ATL carriers [41]. Ishigaki et al. [32] established the four-color flow cytometry system to distinguish HTLV-1 carriers with a high risk for ATL development from those with a low risk, by selecting the CADM1 versus CD7 plot [32].

### 3.3.4 Provirus Load

A higher HTLV-1 provirus DNA load in the peripheral blood mononuclear cells (PBMCs) is a strong risk marker for developing ATL from asymptomatic HTLV-1 carriers [26, 33, 45, 56]. In particular, HTLV-1 carriers with a high provirus load >4 copies/100 PBMCs is an independent factor for progression of ATL, even after adjusting for sex, age, family history of ATL, and other possible risk factors [33]. Nevertheless, the association between HTLV-1 provirus load and disease development remains unclear because the majority of HTLV-1 carriers with a higher provirus load remain ATL-free, and a higher HTLV-1 provirus load is also an important predictor for the development of HAM/TSP.

### 3.3.5 Provirus Integration Status

Some HTLV-1 carriers have monoclonal integration of HTLV-1 provirus DNA into mononuclear cells, without signs of malignant proliferation or clinical signs and symptoms related to leukemia [30]. Such carriers are suggested to be a high-risk group for development of ATL, but their prognosis varies from being stable long-term carriers to development of ATL [30, 31]. Carvalho and Da Fonseca Porto [10] also found a correlation between monoclonal integration of provirus DNA and abnormal lymphocytes in peripheral blood, with a trend for greater severity of the parasitic infection.

## 3.4 Transmission of HTLV-1 and Its Prevention

Direct cell-to-cell contact is required for the efficient transmission of HTLV-1 [6]. There are three main routes of transmission of HTLV-1: mother to child via breastfeeding [22], sexual intercourse [37], and blood transfusions containing cellular blood components [57]. Other minor modes of transmission are parenteral transmission via needle-sharing among drug users and via organ transplantation from HTLV-1-infected donors.

### 3.4.1 *Mother-to-Child Transmission and Its Prevention*

Intrauterine transmission via transplacental infection or placental micro-transfusion is rare because no provirus HTLV-1 DNA was detected in cord blood of infected mothers [38]. Instead, postnatal transmission via breastfeeding is the major route of mother-to-child transmission [22]. Gender difference in the transmission rate via breastfeeding is debatable [91]. The major risk factors for HTLV-1 transmission via breastfeeding from mother to child are long duration of breastfeeding for >6 months, high HTLV-1 antibody titers in maternal serum, and high level of HTLV-1 provirus load in breast milk [47, 91].

As ATL and HAM develop only from HTLV-1 carriers and most HTLV-1 infection results from mother-to-child transmission, prevention of transmission via breastfeeding is the most efficient way to reduce the development of HTLV-1-associated diseases. Since the discovery of breastfeeding transmission in 1985 in Japan, several interventional programs to prevent breastfeeding transmission have been implemented. The most active prefecture-wide intervention program, named the ATL Prevention Program, was started in August 1987 in Nagasaki [23]. The efficiency of the program showed that the transmission rate was 2.4% when there was no breastfeeding, 8.3% when breastfeeding was limited to <6 months, and 20% when breastfeeding was >6 months [22]. In Jamaica, a prospective study showed that 32% of children breastfed for >12 months were infected, compared with 9% of those breastfed for <12 months [93].

### 3.4.2 *Sexual Transmission and Its Prevention*

Sexual transmission is the second main route of HTLV-1 transmission. Sexual transmission occurs predominantly from male to female via HTLV-1-infected lymphocytes in semen [48]. A prospective cohort study in Japan reported that the rate of transmission was 3.9 times higher if the carrier spouse was male rather than female [74]. A recent retrospective cohort analysis of new HTLV-1 infections of HTLV-1-negative repeat blood donors also reported that the incidence of new

HTLV-1 positivity was 3 times higher in female donors than male donors [67]. These are thought to be responsible for the increased HTLV-1 seroprevalence with age in female blood donors than in male donors after age 30 years [66]. The efficiency of male-to-female transmission of HTLV-1 is thought to depend on viral load and duration of married life [37, 72]. Therefore, contraceptive use is the only preventive measure for sexual transmission of HTLV-1.

### *3.4.3 Blood-Borne Transmission and Its Prevention*

Transmission of HTLV-1 through blood transfusion was verified serologically and virologically in Japan [57, 68]. Retrospective analyses of HTLV-1-negative recipients who were transfused with blood positive for HTLV-1 antibody found that 62% of recipients had seroconverted [57]. To prevent virus transmission via blood transfusion, countrywide serological screening of donated blood for HTLV-1 has been implemented in Japan, followed by the USA in 1988, France in 1991, Brazil in 1993, and the UK in 2002. In Japan, HTLV-1 transmission via transfusion has been almost eliminated through the serological screening of donated blood using the particle agglutination assay (until 2007) and chemiluminescence enzyme immunoassay since 2008 and indirect immunofluorescence assay as a confirmatory test for screening test-positive blood [66].

Transmission of HTLV-1 through needle-sharing is another route of blood-borne transmission. No data are available for this transmission route in Japan. In Brazil and Latin America, several reports show an increasing number of new HTLV-1 infections through needle-sharing with the length of the needle use [19]. As with HIV prevention, public education, such as needle exchange programs, is the only way to prevent new transmission.

Furthermore, there are a non-negligible number of case reports about transmission of HTLV-1 through organ transplantation from HTLV-1-positive donors to HTLV-1-negative recipients, with subsequent development of HAM [5, 53, 85]. To prevent new transmission via organ transplantation, prior screening of the donor's HTLV-1 status should be mandatory.

## 3.5 Future Perspective

Strategies for prevention of mother-to-child and blood transfusion transmission of HTLV-1 have reduced the number of new infections. Advanced biological techniques have revealed many molecular mechanisms and risk factors for the development of ATL in HTLV-1 carriers. However, there is still no strategy to eliminate HTLV-1 from infected individuals or to prevent ATL development from the virus carrier status. The ultimate preventive and therapeutic strategy is a vaccine to eliminate or neutralize HTLV-1 infection or to prevent the development of ATL and HAM in asymptomatic HTLV-1 carriers. Several vaccine designs have been developed, such as HTLV-1 Tax DNA-targeted vaccine [54] and HTLV peptide-based vaccine [40, 77]. Recently, additional promising vaccines and antibodies have been developed, such as dendritic cell-based anti-HTLV-1 vaccine [64, 75], anti-HBZ vaccine [76], and antibodies against envelope gp46 [80].

## References

1. Abbaszadegan MR, Gholamin M, Tabatabaee A, Farid R, Houshmand M, Abbaszadegan M. Prevalence of human T-lymphotropic virus type 1 among blood donors from Mashhad, Iran. J Clin Microbiol. 2003;41:2593–5.
2. Ades AE, Parker S, Walker J, Edginton M, Taylor GP, Weber JN. Human T-cell Leukaemia/lymphoma virus infection in pregnant women in the United Kingdom: population study. BMJ. 2000;320:1497–501.
3. Aoki R, Karube K, Sugita Y, Nomura Y, Shimizu K, Kimura Y, Hashikawa K, Suefuji N, Kikuchi M, Ohshima K. Distribution of malignant lymphoma in Japan: analysis of 2260 cases, 2001–2006. Pathol Int. 2008;58:174–82.
4. Arisawa K, Soda M, Endo S, Kurokawa K, Katamine S, Shimokawa I, Koba T, Takahashi T, Saito H, Doi H, Shirahama S. Evaluation of adult T-cell leukemia/lymphoma incidence and its impact on non-Hodgkin lymphoma incidence in southwestern Japan. Int J Cancer. 2000;85:319–24.
5. Armstrong MJ, Corbett C, Rowe IA, Taylor GP, Neuberger JM. HTLV-1 in solid-organ transplantation: current challenges and future management strategies. Transplantation. 2012;94:1075–84.
6. Bangham CR. The immune control and cell-to-cell spread of human T-lymphotropic virus type 1. J Gen Virol. 2003;84:3177–89.
7. Birmann BM, Breen EC, Stuver S, Cranston B, Martínez-Maza O, Falk KI, Okayama A, Hanchard B, Mueller N, Hisada M. Population differences in immune marker profiles associated with human T-cell leukemia virus type I infection in Japan and Jamaica. Int J Cancer. 2009;124:614–21.
8. Bittencourt AL, Oliveira PD, Bittencourt VG, Carvalho EM, Farre L. Adult T-cell leukemia/lymphoma triggered by adalimumab. J Clin Virol. 2013;58:494–6.
9. Carneiro-Proietti AB, Sabino EC, Leão S, Salles NA, Loureiro P, Sarr M, Wright D, Busch M, Proietti FA, Murphy EL, NHLBI Retrovirus Epidemiology Donor Study-II (Reds-II), International Component. Human T-lymphotropic virus type 1 and type 2 seroprevalence, incidence, and residual transfusion risk among blood donors in Brazil during 2007–2009. AIDS Res Hum Retrovir. 2012;28:1265–72.
10. Carvalho EM, Da Fonseca PA. Epidemiological and clinical interaction between HTLV-1 and Strongyloides stercoralis. Parasite Immunol. 2004;26:487–97.
11. Chang YB, Kaidarova Z, Hindes D, Bravo M, Kiely N, Kamel H, Dubay D, Hoose B, Murphy EL. Seroprevalence and demographic determinants of human T-lymphotropic virus type 1 and 2 infections among first-time blood donors–United States, 2000–2009. J Infect Dis. 2014;209:523–31.
12. Chihara D, Ito H, Katanoda K, Shibata A, Matsuda T, Tajima K, Sobue T, Matsuo K. Increase in incidence of adult T-cell leukemia/lymphoma in non-endemic areas of Japan and the United States. Cancer Sci. 2012;103:1857–60.
13. de Thé G, Bomford R. An HTLV-I vaccine: why, how, for whom? AIDS Res Hum Retrovir. 1993;9:381–6.

14. Einsiedel L, Verdonck K, Gotuzzo E. Human T-lymphotropic virus 1: clinical aspects of a neglected infection among indigenous populations. In: Scheld WM, Grayson ML, Hughes JM, editors. Emerging infections. 9th ed. Washington, DC: ASM Press; 2010.
15. Fritz A, Percy C, Jack A, Shanmugaratnam K, Sobin L, Parkin DM, Whelan S. International classification of diseases for oncology. 3rd ed. Geneva: World Health Organization; 2000.
16. Gabet AS, Mortreux F, Talarmin A, Plumelle Y, Leclercq I, Leroy A, Gessain A, Clity E, Joubert M, Wattel E. High circulating proviral load with oligoclonal expansion of HTLV-1 bearing T cells in HTLV-1 carriers with strongyloidiasis. Oncogene. 2000;19:4954–60.
17. Gessain A. Epidemiology of HTLV-I and associated diseases. In: Hollsberg P, Hafler DA, editors. Human T-cell lymphotropic virus type 1. Chichester: Wiley; 1996. p. 33–64.
18. Gessain A, Cassar O. Epidemiological aspects and world distribution of HTLV-1 infection. Front Microbiol. 2012;3:388.
19. Gotuzzo E, Arango C, de Queiroz-Campos A, Istúriz RE. Human T-cell lymphotropic virus-I in Latin America. Infect Dis Clin N Am. 2000;14:211–39.
20. Hanchard B. Adult T-cell leukemia/lymphoma in Jamaica: 1986–1995. J Acquir Immune Defic Syndr Hum Retrovirol. 1996;13:S20–5.
21. Hattori T, Uchiyama T, Toibana T, Takatsuki K, Uchino H. Surface phenotype of Japanese adult T-cell leukemia cells characterized by monoclonal antibodies. Blood. 1981;58:645–7.
22. Hino S. Establishment of the milk-borne transmission as akey factor for the peculiar endemicity of humanT-lymphotropic virus type1 (HTLV-1): the ATL prevention program Nagasaki. Proc Jpn Acad Ser B Phys Biol Sci. 2011;87:152–66.
23. Hino S, Sugiyama H, Doi H, Ishimaru T, Yamabe T, Tsuji Y, Miyamoto T. Breaking the cycle of HTLV-I transmission via carrier mothers' milk. Lancet. 1987;2:158–9.
24. Hinuma Y, Komoda H, Chosa T, Kondo T, Kohakura M, Takenaka T, Kikuchi M, Ichimaru M, Yunoki K, Sato I, Matsuo R, Takiuchi Y, Uchino H, Hanaoka M. Antibodies to adult T-cell leukemia-virus-associated antigen (ATLA) in sera from patients with ATL and controls in Japan: a nation-wide sero-epidemiologic study. Int J Cancer. 1982;29:631–5.
25. Hinuma Y, Nagata K, Hanaoka M, Nakai M, Matsumoto T, Kinoshita D, Shirakawa S, Miyoshi I. Adult T cell leukemia: antigen in an ATL cell line and detection of antibodies to the antigen in human sera. Proc Natl Acad Sci U S A. 1981;78:6476–80.
26. Hisada M, Okayama A, Shioiri S, Spiegelman DL, Stuver SO, Mueller NE. Risk factors for adult T-cell leukemia among carriers of human T-lymphotropic virus type I. Blood. 1998;92:3557–61.
27. Hisada M, Okayama A, Spiegelman D, Mueller NE, Stuver SO. Sex-specific mortality from adult T-cell leukemia among carriers of human T-lymphotropic virus type I. Int J Cancer. 2001;91:497–9.
28. Hoshida Y, Li T, Dong Z, Tomita Y, Yamauchi A, Hanai J, Aozasa K. Lymphoproliferative disorders in renal transplant patients in Japan. Int J Cancer. 2001;91:869–75.
29. IARC. Human immunodeficiency viruses and human T-cell lymphotropic viruses. IARC Monogr Eval Carcinog Risks Hum. 1996;67:1–424.
30. Ikeda S, Momita S, Kinoshita K, et al. Clinical course of human T-lymphotropic virus type I carriers with molecularly detectable monoclonal proliferation of T lymphocytes: defining a low- and high-risk population. Blood. 1993;82:2017.
31. Imaizumi Y, Iwanaga M, Tsukasaki K, Hata T, Tomonaga M, Ikeda S. Natural course of HTLV-1 carriers with monoclonal proliferation of T lymphocytes ("pre-ATL") in a 20-year follow-up study. Blood. 2005;105:903–4.
32. Ishigaki T, Zaike Y, Nojima M, Kobayashi S, Ohno N, Uchimaru K, Tojo A, Nakauchi H, Watanabe N. Quantification of adult T-cell leukemia/lymphoma cells using simple four-color flow cytometry. Clin Chem Lab Med. 2015;53:85–93.
33. Iwanaga M, Watanabe T, Utsunomiya A, Okayama A, Uchimaru K, Koh KR, Ogata M, Kikuchi H, Sagara Y, Uozumi K, Mochizuki M, Tsukasaki K, Saburi Y, Yamamura M, Tanaka J, Moriuchi Y, Hino S, Kamihira S, Yamaguchi K, Joint Study on Predisposing Factors of ATL Development investigators. Human T-cell leukemia virus type I (HTLV-1) proviral

load and disease progression in asymptomatic HTLV-1 carriers: a nationwide prospective study in Japan. Blood. 2010;116:1211–9.
34. Iwanaga M, Watanabe T, Yamaguchi K. Adult T-cell leukemia: a review of epidemiological evidence. Front Microbiol. 2012;3:322.
35. Kamihira S, Atogami S, Sohda H, Momita S, Yamada Y, Tomonaga M. Significance of soluble interleukin-2 receptor levels for evaluation of the progression of adult T-cell leukemia. Cancer. 1994;73:2753–8.
36. Kamihira S, Iwanaga M, Doi Y, Sasaki D, Mori S, Tsurda K, Nagai K, Uno N, Hasegawa H, Yanagihara K, Morinaga Y, Tsukasaki K, Taniguchi H. Heterogeneity in clonal nature in the smoldering subtype of adult T-cell leukemia: continuity from carrier status to smoldering ATL. Int J Hematol. 2012;95:399–408.
37. Kaplan JE, Khabbaz RF, Murphy EL, Hermansen S, Roberts C, Lal R, Heneine W, Wright D, Matijas L, Thomson R, Rudolph D, Switzer WM, Kleinman S, Busch M, Schreiber GB. Male-to-female transmission of human T-cell lymphotropic virus types I and II: association with viral load. The Retrovirus Epidemiology Donor Study Group. J Acquir Immune Defic Syndr Hum Retrovirol. 1996;12:193–201.
38. Katamine S, Moriuchi R, Yamamoto T, Terada K, Eguchi K, Tsuji Y, Yamabe T, Miyamoto T, Hino S. HTLV-I proviral DNA in umbilical cord blood of babies born to carrier mothers. Lancet. 1994;343:1326–7.
39. Kawano N, Shimoda K, Ishikawa F, Taketomi A, Yoshizumi T, Shimoda S, Yoshida S, Uozumi K, Suzuki S, Maehara Y, Harada M. Adult T-cell leukemia development from a human T-cell leukemia virus type I carrier after a living-donor liver transplantation. Transplantation. 2006;82:840–3.
40. Kazanji M, Heraud JM, Merien F, Pique C, de Thé G, Gessain A, Jacobson S. Chimeric peptide vaccine composed of B- and T-cell epitopes of human T-cell leukemia virus type 1 induces humoral and cellular immune responses and reduces the proviral load in immunized squirrel monkeys (*Saimiri sciureus*). J Gen Virol. 2006;87:1331–7.
41. Kobayashi S, Nakano K, Watanabe E, Ishigaki T, Ohno N, Yuji K, Oyaizu N, Asanuma S, Yamagishi M, Yamochi T, Watanabe N, Tojo A, Watanabe T, Uchimaru K. CADM1 expression and stepwise downregulation of CD7 are closely associated with clonal expansion of HTLV-1-infected cells in adult T-cell leukemia/lymphoma. Clin Cancer Res. 2014;20:2851–61.
42. Koga Y, Iwanaga M, Soda M, Inokuchi N, Sasaki D, Hasegawa H, Yanagihara K, Yamaguchi K, Kamihira S, Yamada Y. Trends in HTLV-1 prevalence and the incidence of adult Tcell leukemia/lymphoma (ATLL) in Nagasaki, Japan. J Med Virol. 2010;82:668–74.
43. Laperche S, Worms B, Pillonel J, European Network of Transfusion Medecine Societies, Steering Committee. Blood safety strategies for human T-cell lymphotropic virus in Europe. Vox Sang. 2009;96:104–10.
44. Levine PH, Dosik H, Joseph EM, Felton S, Bertoni MA, Cervantes J, Moulana V, Miotti AB, Goberdhan LJ, Lee SL, Daouad A, DaCosta M, Jaffe ES, Axiotis CA, Cleghorn FR, Kahn A, Welles SL. A study of adult T-cell leukemia/lymphoma incidence in central Brooklyn. Int J Cancer. 1999;80:662–6.
45. Manns A, Miley WJ, Wilks RJ, Morgan OS, Hanchard B, Wharfe G, Cranston B, Maloney E, Welles SL, Blattner WA, Waters D. Quantitative proviral DNA and antibody levels in the natural history of HTLV-1 infection. J Infect Dis. 1999;180:1487–93.
46. Matsuoka M, Jeang KT. Human T-cell leukemia virus type 1 (HTLV-1) and leukemic transformation: viral infectivity, Tax, HBZ and therapy. Oncogene. 2011;30:1379–89.
47. Moriuchi H, Masuzaki H, Doi H, Katamine S. Mother-to-child transmission of human T-cell lymphotropic virus type 1. Pediatr Infect Dis J. 2013;32:175–7.
48. Murphy EL, Figueroa JP, Gibbs WN, Brathwaite A, Holding-Cobham M, Waters D, Cranston B, Hanchard B, Blattner WA. Sexual transmission of human T-lymphotropic virus type I (HTLV-I). Ann Intern Med. 1989b;111:555–60.

49. Murphy EL, Figueroa JP, Gibbs WN, Holding-Cobham M, Cranston B, Malley K, Bodner AJ, Alexander SS, Blattner WA. Human T-lymphotropic virus type I (HTLV-I) seroprevalence in Jamaica. I. Demographic determinants. Am J Epidemiol. 1991;133:1114–24.
50. Murphy EL, Hanchard B, Figueroa JP, Gibbs WN, Lofters WS, Campbell M, Goedert JJ, Blattner WA. Modelling the risk of adult T-cell leukemia/lymphoma in persons infected with human T-lymphotropic virus type I. Int J Cancer. 1989a;43:250–3.
51. Nakada K, Yamaguchi K, Furugen S, Nakasone T, Nakasone K, Oshiro Y, Kohakura M, Hinuma Y, Seiki M, Yoshida M, Matutes E, Catovsky D, Ishii T, Takatsuki K. Monoclonal integration of HTLV-I proviral DNA in patients with strongyloidiasis. Int J Cancer. 1987;40:145–8.
52. Nakamura H, Ueki Y, Saito S, Horai Y, Suzuki T, Naoe T, Eguchi K, Kawakami A. Development of adult T-cell leukemia in a patient with rheumatoid arthritis treated with tocilizumab. Intern Med. 2013;52:1983–6.
53. Nakatsuji Y, Sugai F, Watanabe S, Kaido M, Koguchi K, Abe K, Sakoda S. HTLV-I-associated myelopathy manifested after renal transplantation. J Neurol Sci. 2000;177:154–6.
54. Ohashi T, Hanabuchi S, Kato H, Tateno H, Takemura F, Tsukahara T, Koya Y, Hasegawa A, Masuda T, Kannagi M. Prevention of adult T-cell leukemia-like lymphoproliferative disease in rats by adoptively transferred T cells from a donor immunized with human T-cell leukemia virus type 1 Tax-coding DNA vaccine. J Virol. 2000;74:9610–6.
55. Ohshima K, Suzumiya J, Kikuchi M. The World Health Organization classification of malignant lymphoma: incidence and clinical prognosis in HTLV-1-endemic area of Fukuoka. Pathol Int. 2002;52:1–12.
56. Okayama A, Stuver S, Matsuoka M, Ishizaki J, Tanaka G, Kubuki Y, Mueller N, Hsieh CC, Tachibana N, Tsubouchi H. Role of HTLV-1 proviral DNA load and clonality in the development of adult T-cell leukemia/lymphoma in asymptomatic carriers. Int J Cancer. 2004;110:621–5.
57. Okochi K, Sato H, Hinuma Y. A retrospective study on transmission of adult T cell leukemia virus by blood transfusion: seroconversion in recipients. Vox Sang. 1984;46:245–53.
58. Paun L, Ispas O, Del Mistro A, Chieco-Bianchi L. HTLV-I in Romania. Eur J Haematol. 1994;52:117–8.
59. Poiesz BJ, Ruscetti FW, Gazdar AF, Bunn PA, Minna JD, Gallo RC. Detection and isolation of type C retrovirus particles from fresh and cultured lymphocytes of a patient with cutaneous T-cell lymphoma. Proc Natl Acad Sci U S A. 1980;77:7415–9.
60. Pombo-de-Oliveira MS, Loureiro P, Bittencourt A, Chiattone C, Borducchi D, De Carvalho SM, Barbosa HS, Rios M, Sill A, Cleghorn F, Blattner W. Geographic diversity of adult t-cell leukemia/lymphoma in Brazil. The Brazilian ATLL Study Group. Int J Cancer. 1999;83:291–8.
61. Pombo-de-Oliveira MS, Matutes E, Schulz T, Carvalho SM, Noronha H, Reaves JD, Loureiro P, Machado C, Catovsky D. T-cell malignancies in Brazil: clinico-pathological and molecular studies of HTLV-I positive and negative cases. Int J Cancer. 1995;60:823–7.
62. Proietti FA, Carneiro-Proietti AB, Catalan-Soares BC, Murphy EL. Global epidemiology of HTLV-I infection and associated diseases. Oncogene. 2005;24:6058–68.
63. Rafatpanah H, Hedayati-Moghaddam MR, Fathimoghadam F, Bidkhori HR, Shamsian SK, Ahmadi S, Bazarbachi A. High prevalence of HTLV-I infection in Mashhad, Northeast Iran: a population-based seroepidemiology survey. J Clin Virol. 2011;52:172–6.
64. Sagar D, Masih S, Schell T, Jacobson S, Wigdahl B, Khan Z, Jain P. In vivo immunogenicity of Tax 11-19 epitope in HLA-A2/DTR transgenic mice: implication for dendritic cell-based anti-HTLV-1 vaccine (VAC12P. 1020). J Immunol. 2014;192(Supplement):206–9.
65. Satake M, Yamada Y, Atogami S, Yamaguchi K. The incidence of adult T-cell leukemia/lymphoma among human T-lymphotropic virus type 1 carriers in Japan. Leuk Lymphoma. 2015;56:1806–12.
66. Satake M, Yamaguchi K, Tadokoro K. Current prevalence of HTLV-1 in Japan as determined by screening of blood donors. J Med Virol. 2012;84:327–35.

67. Satake M, Iwanaga M, Sagara Y, Watanabe T, Okuma K, Hamaguchi I. Incidence of human T-lymphotropic virus 1 infection in adolescent and adult blood donors in Japan: a nationwide retrospective cohort analysis. Lancet Infect Dis. 2016;16:1246–54.
68. Sato H, Okochi K. Transmission of human T-cell leukemia virus (HTLV-I) by blood transfusion: demonstration of proviral DNA in recipients' blood lymphocytes. Int J Cancer. 1986;37:395–400.
69. Satoh M, Toma H, Sugahara K, Etoh K, Shiroma Y, Kiyuna S, Takara M, Matsuoka M, Yamaguchi K, Nakada K, Fujita K, Kojima S, Hori E, Tanaka Y, Kamihira S, Sato Y, Watanabe T. Involvement of IL-2/IL-2R system activation by parasite antigen in polyclonal expansion of CD4(+)25(+) HTLV-1-infected T-cells in human carriers of both HTLV-1 and S. stercoralis. Oncogene. 2002;21:2466–75.
70. Schreiber GB, Murphy EL, Horton JA, Wright DJ, Garfein R, Chien HC, Nass CC. Risk factors for human T-cell lymphotropic virus types I and II (HTLV-I and -II) in blood donors: the Retrovirus Epidemiology Donor Study. NHLBI Retrovirus Epidemiology Donor Study. J Acquir Immune Defic Syndr Hum Retrovirol. 1997;14:263–71.
71. Shimoyama M. Diagnostic criteria and classification of clinical subtypes of adult T-cell leukaemia-lymphoma:a report from the Lymphoma Study Group (1984–87). Br J Haematol. 1991;79:428–37.
72. Shirley MH, Sayeed S, Barnes I, Finlayson A, Ali R. Incidence of haematological malignancies by ethnic group in England, 2001-7. Br J Haematol. 2013;163:465–77.
73. Sonoda S, Li HC, Tajima K. Ethnoepidemiology of HTLV-1 related diseases: ethnic determinants of HTLV-1 susceptibility and its worldwide dispersal. Cancer Sci. 2011;102:295–301.
74. Stuver SO, Tachibana N, Okayama A, Shioiri S, Tsunetoshi Y, Tsuda K, Mueller NE. Heterosexual transmission of human T cell leukemia/lymphoma virus type I among married couples in southwestern Japan: an initial report from the Miyazaki cohort study. J Infect Dis. 1993;167:57–65.
75. Suehiro Y, Hasegawa A, Iino T, Sasada A, Watanabe N, Matsuoka M, Takamori A, Tanosaki R, Utsunomiya A, Choi I, Fukuda T, Miura O, Takaishi S, Teshima T, Akashi K, Kannagi M, Uike N, Okamura J. Clinical outcomes of a novel therapeutic vaccine with Tax peptide-pulsed dendritic cells for adult T cell leukaemia/lymphoma in a pilot study. Br J Haematol. 2015;169:356–67.
76. Sugata K, Yasunaga JI, Mitobe Y, Miura M, Miyazato P, Kohara M, Matsuoka M. Protective effect of cytotoxic T lymphocytes targeting HTLV-1 bZIP factor. Blood. 2015;126 (9):1095–105.
77. Sundaram R, Lynch MP, Rawale SV, Sun Y, Kazanji M, Kaumaya PT. De novo design of peptide immunogens that mimic the coiled coil region of human T-cell leukemia virus type-1 glycoprotein 21 transmembrane subunit for induction of native protein reactive neutralizing antibodies. J Biol Chem. 2004;279:24141–51.
78. Tajima K. The 4th nation-wide study of adult T-cell leukemia/lymphoma (ATL) in Japan: estimates of risk of ATL and its geographical and clinical features. The T- and B-cell Malignancy Study Group. Int J Cancer. 1990;45:237–43.
79. Takatsuki K, Uchiyama J, Sagawa K, Yodoi J. Adult T-cell leukemia in Japan. In: Seno S, Takaku F, Irino S, editors. Topics in hematology. Amsterdam: Excerpta Medica; 1977. p. 73–7.
80. Tanaka Y, Takahashi Y, Tanaka R, Kodama A, Fujii H, Hasegawa A, Kannagi M, Ansari AA, Saito M. Elimination of human T cell leukemia virus type-1-infected cells by neutralizing and antibody-dependent cellular cytotoxicity-inducing antibodies against human t cell leukemia virus type-1 envelope gp46. AIDS Res Hum Retrovir. 2014;30:542–52.
81. The T- and B-Cell Malignancy Study Group. Statistical analyses of clinico-pathological, virological and epidemiological data on lymphoid malignancies with special reference to adult T-cell leukemia/lymphoma: a report of the second nationwide study of Japan. Jpn J Clin Oncol. 1985;15:517–35.
82. The T- and B-cell malignancy Study Group. The 9th nation-wide study of adult T-cell leukemia/lymphoma (ATL) in Japan. Gan No Rinsho. 2001;47:341–57. [Japanese]

83. Tian Y, Kobayashi S, Ohno N, Isobe M, Tsuda M, Zaike Y, Watanabe N, Tani K, Tojo A, Uchimaru K. Leukemic T cells are specifically enriched in a unique CD3(dim) CD7(low) subpopulation of CD4(+) T cells in acute-type adult T-cell leukemia. Cancer Sci. 2011;102:569–77.
84. Tokudome S, Tokunaga O, Shimamoto Y, Miyamoto Y, Sumida I, Kikuchi M, Takeshita M, Ikeda T, Fujiwara K, Yoshihara M, Yanagawa T, Nishizumi M. Incidence of adult T-cell leukemia/lymphoma among human T-lymphotropic virus type I carriers in Saga, Japan. Cancer Res. 1989;49:226–8.
85. Toro C, Rodes B, Poveda E, Soriano (2003) Rapid development of subacute myelopathy in three organ transplant recipients after transmission of human T-cell lymphotropic virus type I from a single donor. Transplantation 75:102–104.
86. Treviño A, Vicario JL, Lopez M, Parra P, Benito R, Ortiz de Lejarazu R, Ramos JM, Del Romero J, de Mendoza C, Soriano V. Association between HLA alleles and HAM/TSP in individuals infected with HTLV-1. J Neurol. 2013;60:2551–5.
87. Tsuji T, Sugahara K, Tsuruda K, Uemura A, Harasawa H, Hasegawa H, Hamaguchi Y, Tomonaga M, Yamada Y, Kamihira S. Clinical and oncologic implications in epigenetic down-regulation of CD26/dipeptidyl peptidase IV in adult T-cell leukemia cells. Int J Hematol. 2004;80:254–60.
88. Tsurumi H, Tani K, Tsuruta T, Shirato R, Matsudaira T, Tojo A, Wada C, Uchida H, Ozawa K, Asano S. Adult T-cell leukemia developing during immunosuppressive treatment in a renal transplant recipient. Am J Hematol. 1992;41:292–4.
89. Uchiyama T, Yodoi J, Sagawa K, Takatsuki K, Uchino H. Adult T-cell leukemia: clinical and hematologic features of 16 cases. Blood. 1977;50:481–92.
90. Uno H, Kawano K, Matsuoka H, Tsuda K. HLA and adult T-cell leukaemia: HLA-linked genes controlling susceptibility to human T-cell leukaemia vims type I. Clin Exp Immunol. 1988;71:211–5.
91. Ureta-Vidal A, Angelin-Duclos C, Tortevoye P, Murphy E, Lepère JF, Buigues RP, Jolly N, Joubert M, Carles G, Pouliquen JF, de Thé G, Moreau JP, Gessain A. Mother-to-child transmission of human T-cell-leukemia/lymphoma virus type I: implication of high antiviral antibody titer and high proviral load in carrier mothers. Int J Cancer. 1999;82:832–6.
92. Verdonck K, Gonzalez E, Van Dooren S, Vandamme AM, Vanham G, Vanham G, Gotuzzo E. Human T-lymphotropic virus 1: recent knowledge about an ancient infection. Lancet Infect Dis. 2007;7:266–81.
93. Wiktor SZ, Pate EJ, Rosenberg PS, Barnett M, Palmer P, Medeiros D, Maloney EM, Blattner WA. Motherto- child transmission of human T-cell lymphotropic virus type I associated with prolonged breast-feeding. J Hum Virol. 1997;1:37–44.
94. Yamada Y, Atogami S, Hasegawa H, Kamihira S, Soda M, Satake M, Yamaguchi K. Nationwide survey of adult T-cell leukemia/lymphoma (ATL) in Japan. Rinsho Ketsueki. 2011;52:1765–71. [Japanese]
95. Yamaguchi K, Seiki M, Yoshida M, Nishimura H, Kawano F, Takatsuki K. The detection of human T cell leukemia virus proviral DNA and its application for classification and diagnosis of T cell malignancy. Blood. 1984;63:1235–40.
96. Yamamoto JF, Goodman MT. Patterns of leukemia incidence in the United States by subtype and demographic characteristics, 1997–2002. Cancer Causes Control. 2008;19:379–90.
97. Yashiki S, Fujiyoshi T, Arima N, Osame M, Yoshinaga M, Nagata Y, Tara M, Nomura K, Utsunomiya A, Hanada S, Tajima K, Sonoda S. HLA-A*26, HLA-B*4002, HLAB*4006, and HLA-B* 4801 alleles predispose to adult T cell leukemia: the limited recognition of HTLV type 1 tax peptide anchor motifs and epitopes to generate anti-HTLV type 1 tax CD8(+) cytotoxic T lymphocytes. AIDS Res Hum Retrovir. 2001;17:1047–61.
98. Yoshida M, Miyoshi I, Hinuma Y. Isolation and characterization of retrovirus from cell lines of human adult T-cell leukemia and its implication in the disease. Proc Natl Acad Sci U S A. 1982;79:2031–5.
99. Yoshizumi T, Shirabe K, Ikegami T, Kayashima H, Yamashita N, Morita K, Masuda T, Hashimoto N, Taketomi A, Soejima Y, Maehara Y. Impact of human T cell leukemia virus type 1 in living donor liver transplantation. Am J Transplant. 2012;12:1479–85.

# Chapter 4
# Pathology

**Koichi Ohshima and Hiroaki Miyoshi**

## 4.1 Neoplastic Lesions

### *4.1.1 Sites of Involvement*

Most Adult T-cell leukemia/lymphoma (ATL) patients present with widespread lymph node involvement as well as peripheral blood. The fact that the concentration of neoplastic cells in a peripheral blood sample does not correlate with the degree of bone marrow involvement suggests that circulating neoplastic cells are recruited from other organs such as the skin and lymph nodes, and indeed, the skin is the most common extralymphatic site of involvement (>50% of patients with ATL) [7]. Other clinically relevant extranodal sites of involvement associated with morbidity include the lungs, liver, spleen, gastrointestinal tract, and central nervous system [8] (Table 4.1).

### *4.1.2 Clinical Features: Peripheral Blood*

Four clinical subtypes of ATL have been identified: acute, lymphomatous, chronic, and smoldering (Table 4.2) [9]. Because most patients have stage IV disease at presentation, the Ann Arbor staging system is not prognostically useful. The most common subtypes, acute ATL, is characterized by a leukemic phase, often with a markedly elevated white blood cell count, skin rash, and generalized lymphadenopathy. The leukemic cells are medium- to large-sized lymphoid cells with

K. Ohshima (✉) • H. Miyoshi
Department of Pathology, School of Medicine, Kurume University, Asahimati 67, Kurume 830-0011, Japan
e-mail: ohshima_kouichi@med.kurume-u.ac.jp



T. Watanabe, T. Fukushima (eds.), *Adult T-cell Leukemia/Lymphoma*,
DOI 10.1007/978-4-431-56523-9_4

**Table 4.1** Human T-cell leukemia virus type I (HTLV-1)-related disease

| **Neoplastic disorders** | **Reactive disorders** |
|---|---|
| Peripheral blood (leukemia) | Confirmed |
| Smoldering type | HTLV-I-associated myelopathy (HAM) |
| Chronic type | HTLV-I-associated uveitis |
| Acute type | Not confirmed |
| Lymph node (Lymphoma) | HTLV-I-associated lymphadenitis |
| Hodgkin's-like type | HTLV-I-associated bronchopneumopathy (HAB) |
| Pleomorphic small-cell type | HTLV-I-associated arthropathy (HAAP) |
| Pleomorphic (medium- and large-cell) type | HTLV-I-associated nephropathy |
| Anaplastic large-cell type | Infective dermatitis |
| Skin | Polymyositis |
| Erythema | Sjögren syndrome |
| Papule | Autoimmune thyroiditis |
| Nodule | Polyneuropathy |
| Tumor | **Immunodeficiency association** |
| Gastrointestinal tract | Strongyloidiasis (gastrointestinal tract) |
| Erosion | Varicella zoster (skin) |
| Ulceration | Crusted scabies (skin) |
| Tumor | Opportunistic lung infection |
| Liver | *Pneumocystis carinii* |
| Portal or sinus infiltration | Cytomegalovirus |
| Bone marrow | Aspergillus fumigatus |
| Infiltration with or without fibrosis | *Candida albicans* |
| Lung | *Cryptococcus neoformans* |
| Interstitial infiltration | Carcinoma (not confirmed) |

Modified from Ref. [64]

**Table 4.2** Diagnostic criteria for clinical subtypes of ATL

| | Smoldering | Chronic | Acute |
|---|---|---|---|
| Lymphocytosis | No | Increased | Increased |
| Blood abnormal lymphocytes | >5% | Increased | Increased |
| LDH | Normal | Slight increased | Increased |
| Ca | Normal | Normal | Variable |
| Skin rash | Erythema, papules | Variable | Variable |
| Lymphadenopathy | No | Mild | Variable |
| Hepatosplenomegaly | No | Mild | Variable |
| Bone marrow infiltration | No | No | Variable |

Modified from Ref. [9]

irregular nuclei and basophilic cytoplasm. Characteristic ATL cells have been described as "flower cells," with many nuclear convolutions and lobules (Fig. 4.1). Patients with ATL usually have hepatosplenomegaly, constitutional symptoms, and elevated lactate dehydrogenase levels. Hypercalcemia, with or

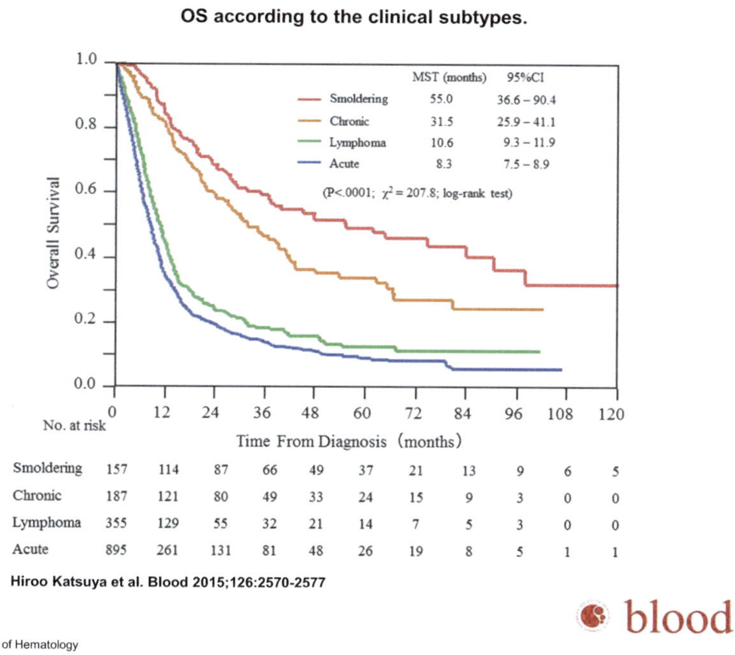


**Fig. 4.1** Survival of patients with ATL subtypes. Acute and lymphomatous forms have an aggressive clinical course, whereas longer survival is seen in patients with chronic or smoldering disease (Adapted from Ref. [9]). In peripheral blood of acute ATL, the leukemic cells are medium-sized to large lymphoid cells with irregular nuclei and basophilic cytoplasm. The characteristic ATL cells have been described as "flower cells" because of their many nuclear convolutions and lobules (**a**). ATL cells in the chronic variant are generally small with slight nuclear abnormalities, such as notching, indentation, and convolution (**b**)

without lytic bone lesions, is a common feature, while leukocytosis and eosinophilia are common complications [10].

The lymphomatous variant is characterized by prominent lymphadenopathy. However, there is no peripheral blood (PB) involvement.

The chronic subtype is associated with skin lesions, most commonly exfoliative. While absolute lymphocytosis may be present, atypical lymphocytes are not numerous in the blood. ATL cells of the chronic subtype are generally small with slightly abnormal notched, indented, and convoluted nuclei (Fig. 4.1). Hypercalcemia is absent. Although patients may have hepatosplenomegaly, the clinical course is generally indolent; the median survival is about 2 years [9].

In patients with the smoldering subtype, the white blood cell count is normal, with >5% circulating neoplastic cells. ATL cells are generally small with a normal appearance of small lymphocyte. Patients frequently have skin or pulmonary lesions and do not have hypercalcemia. Progression from the chronic or smoldering to the acute subtype occurs in 25% of cases, but usually after a long period of time (Fig. 4.1) [9].

### *4.1.3 Lymph Node Lesions*

Histopathological examination of HTLV-I-involved lymph nodes usually, although not uniformly, finds lymph nodes with a typical pleomorphic appearance. In addition to the lymph nodes of patients with overt ATL, the lymph nodes of some patients with pre-ATL show a Hodgkin disease-like morphology. The lymph nodes of carriers without ATL manifest features of lymphadenitis [11–13].

#### 4.1.3.1 Lymphomatous Lesions

##### 4.1.3.1.1 Pleomorphic (Medium- and Large-Cell) Type

The medium and large tumor cells vary in size and show obvious nuclear irregularities. Giant cells with cerebriform, Reed-Sternberg-like or bizarre nuclei are frequently seen in lymph nodes (Fig. 4.2a). This type is the typical nodal lesion of ATL.

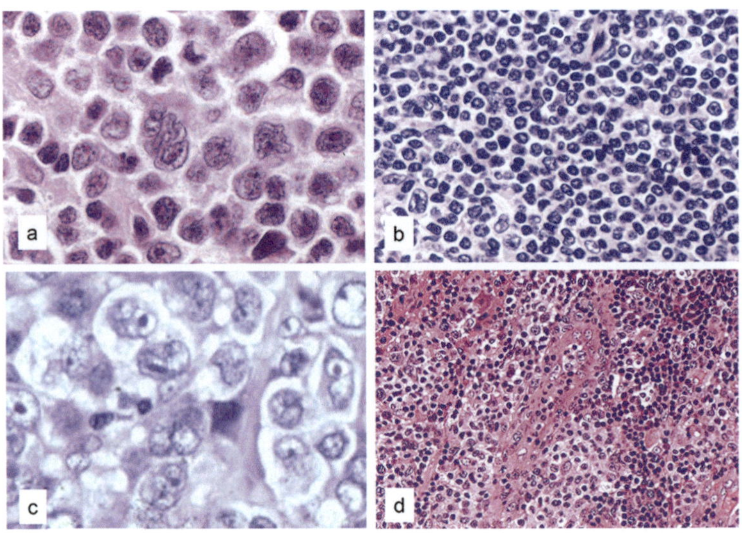


**Fig. 4.2** Histology of HTLV-I associated lymph nodes. (**a**) The pleomorphic (medium-sized and large-cell) type shows a diffuse proliferation of atypical medium-sized to large lymphoid cells with irregular nuclei, intermingled with cerebriform giant cells (*center*). (**b**) The lymph nodes of the pleomorphic small-cell type show a diffuse proliferation of atypical medium-sized to small lymphoid cells. (**c**) The anaplastic large-cell type shows a diffuse proliferation of atypical large lymphoid cells with prominent nucleoli. (**d**) AILT-like ATL shows proliferation of high endothelial venules with a variety of infiltrating inflammatory cells

#### 4.1.3.1.2 Pleomorphic Small-Cell Type

Histologically, these tumor cells are as large as or slightly larger than normal lymphocytes in the peripheral circulation (Fig. 4.2b) and show mild nuclear irregularities, with only a few cells displaying mitotic figures. Tumor cells have the phenotype of a peripheral T cell. [13, 14]

#### 4.1.3.1.3 Anaplastic Large-Cell Type

The tumor cells are much larger than the cells of large-cell lymphoma and show a uniform pattern of cell proliferation. Tumor cells with prominent nucleoli and an abundant cytoplasm have been found, and multinucleated giant cells such as Reed-Sternberg cells have also been detected (Fig. 4.2c). Tumor cells express the CD30 antigen and have the phenotype of a peripheral T cell [13, 15].

#### 4.1.3.1.4 AILT-Like ATL

Angioimmunoblastic T-cell lymphoma (AILT) is a rare morphological variant of ATL. Examined lymph nodes have shown proliferation of high endothelial venules and various infiltrating inflammatory cells, including plasma cells and eosinophils (Fig. 4.2d). The lymphoma cells are medium to large in size, with clear cytoplasm [16].

#### 4.1.3.1.5 Immunophenotypes and Genotypes

Tumor cells express T-cell-associated antigens (CD2, CD3, CD5), but usually not CD7. While the cells of most cases are CD4+CD8-, a few are CD4-CD8+ or double positive/negative for CD4 and CD8. CD25, the interleukin-2 receptor alpha subunit, is strongly expressed in nearly all cases. The large transformed cells may be positive for CD30, but are ALK negative [17]. None of the cases appear to have tumor cells that express the cytotoxic molecules T-cell-restricted intracellular antigen and granzyme B. The absence of the expression of these markers is a key consideration in differentiating between ATL and extranodal cytotoxic T-cell lymphoma in HTLV-I-endemic areas. In addition, tumor cells frequently express the CCR4 chemokine receptor and FoxP3, a regulatory T-cell (Treg) marker [18]. The origin of ATL cells has been postulated to be peripheral CD4+ alpha/beta T cells, and it has been suggested that CD4+CD25+FoxP3+ Treg cells are their closest normal counterpart [18] (Fig. 4.3). The follicular T-cell markers CD10, bcl6, and CXCL13 are not expressed by ATL, including AILT-like ATL, tumor cells.

Most ATL cases are characterized by monoclonal integration of HTLV-I proviral DNA, and some by oligoclonal integration, but clonal integration is not present

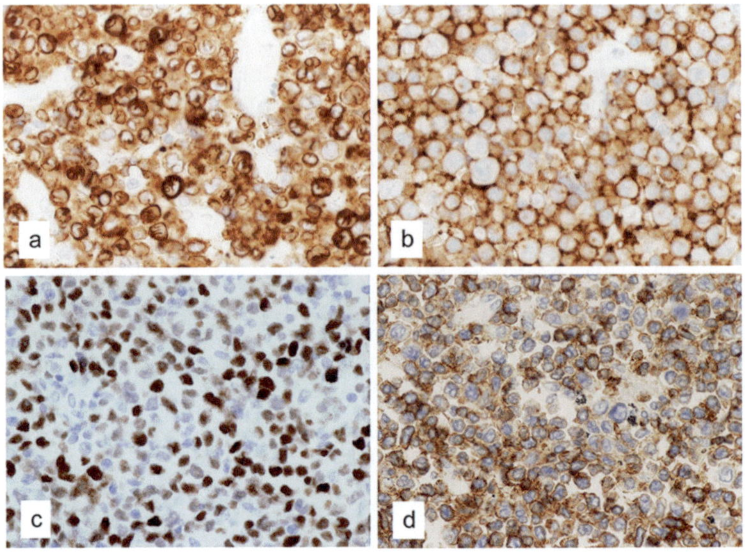


**Fig. 4.3** Immunophenotype of ATL. (**a**) ATL cells express T-cell-associated antigen of CD3 (**a**) and CD4 (**b**). (**c**, **d**) ATL cells frequently express FoxP3 of the regulatory T-cell marker (**c**) and CCR4 of the chemokine receptor (**d**)

in carriers [19]. T-cell receptor genes of the α-, β-, γ-, and δ-chains are clonally rearranged in ATL. While a dominant T-cell clone has not been observed in HTLV-I carriers, oligoclonal T-cell expansion can be detected [19].

### 4.1.3.2 Atypical Lymphomatous and Nonlymphomatous Lesions

#### 4.1.3.2.1 Hodgkin Cell-Like Type

The lymph nodes exhibit a relatively preserved nodal architecture with diffuse infiltration of small- or medium-sized lymphocytes with mild nuclear irregularities. Small aggregated foci or clusters of a few giant cells with irregularly lobulated, highly convoluted, Reed-Sternberg- or Hodgkin cell-like nuclei are scattered throughout the expanded paracortex (Fig. 4.4a). The giant cells occasionally display mitotic features. Immunohistological analysis reveals that proliferating small- to medium-sized lymphocytes possess a peripheral T-cell phenotype of helper/inducer cells (CD1-, CD2+, CD3+, CD4+, CD8-) and that giant cells show a Hodgkin lymphoma phenotype, which reacts with anti-CD30 antibody and/or anti-CD15 and anti-PAX5 antibodies. Analysis of receptor genes has found rearrangement and/or deletion of the T-cell receptor genes Cβ and/or Jγ. Proviral HTLV-I DNA bands have been found, although the bands are weaker than those usually seen in typical ATL, probably because of the small population of integrated HTLV-I lymphocytes. Molecular analysis by single-cell polymerase chain reaction

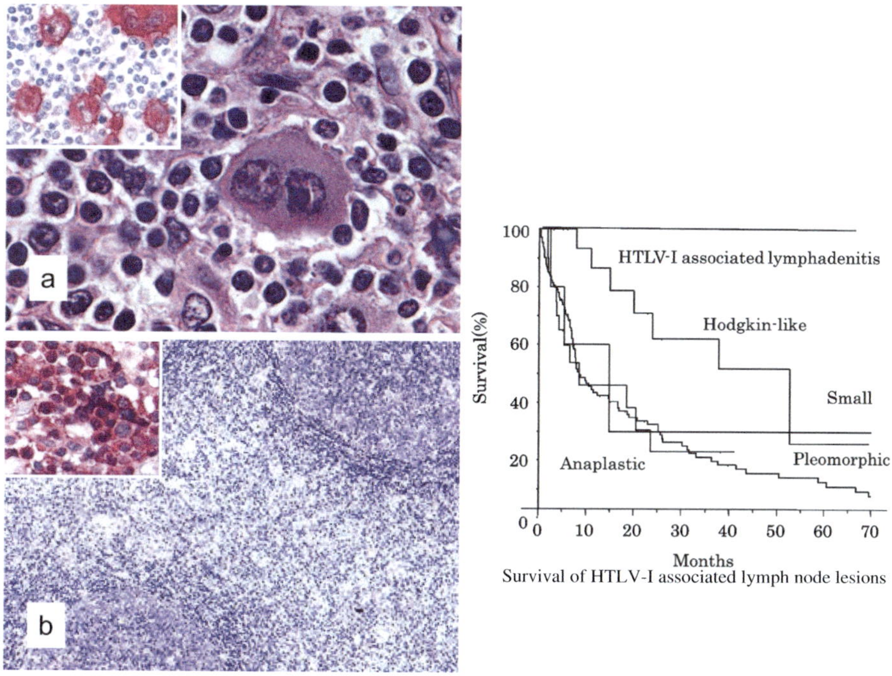


**Fig. 4.4** Survival and histology of HTLV-I associated lymph nodes (Adapted from Ref. [13]). (**a**) The lymph nodes of HTLV-I-associated lymphadenitis show an enlarged paracortex with a diffuse infiltration of lymphocytes, which express the CD4 antigen (*inset*). (**b**) The lymph nodes of Hodgkin-like ATL feature Reed-Sternberg-like giant cells, which react with CD30 antibody (*inset*). Survival curve of HTLV-I-associated lymph node lesions. The pleomorphic (medium- and large-cell) and ALCL types are associated with a rapidly deteriorating survival curve, while Hodgkin's type shows a progressive decline in the survival rate. The pleomorphic small-cell type is associated with an initial steep increase in mortality, which reaches a plateau during the middle and late periods of disease progression. In contrast, all cases with lymphadenitis were still alive at the end of the study concerned (Adapted from Ref. [13])

has confirmed that the giant cells are reactive cells that specifically resemble the immature B cell lineage, while the background CD4-positive T cells, which show evidence of clonality, are HTLV-I infected [11, 20].

#### 4.1.3.2.2 Lymphadenitis Type

Histological examination of the lymph nodes of HTLV-I-associated lymphadenitis shows a preserved nodal architecture with small lymphoid follicles, enlargement of the paracortex, and diffuse infiltration by small- or intermediate-sized lymphocytes (Fig. 4.4b), with the latter cells showing slight nuclear irregularities. Immunohistochemically stained sections have shown proliferating small- to intermediate-sized lymphocytes possessing a peripheral helper/inducer T-cell phenotype (CD1-, CD2+, CD3+, CD4+, CD8-), while no cases have shown rearrangement or deletion of the T-cell receptor genes Cβ and Jγ or rearrangement of the immunoglobulin heavy chain gene (JH). Except for a few cases in which oligoclonal bands were detected, no monoclonal proviral DNA bands have been found. However, these bands were weaker than those of typical ATL cases, probably because of the small population of lymphocytes with integration of HTLV-I proviral DNA [12].

#### 4.1.3.3 Survival Rates

The median survival time (MST) and 2- and 5-year survival rates of patients with the different types of ATL are shown in Fig. 4.3. The survival curve of patients with pleomorphic (medium- and large-cell)-type lesions, which display features typical of ATL, rapidly decreases, during both the early and late stages of the disease (Fig. 4.4). ATL manifested by anaplastic large-cell- and AILT-type lesions is also associated with a highly aggressive course; most patients die within 2 years after diagnosis. ATL with Hodgkin-type lesions was found to be associated with a progressively decreasing survival curve during an observation period of 8 years. Pleomorphic small-cell-type lymphoma has been associated with an initial steep increase in mortality, with plateauing of the rate during the middle and later observation periods. On the other hand, all cases with lymphadenitis were alive at the end of one study (Fig. 4.3) [13].

### *4.1.4 Cutaneous Lesions*

ATL commonly involves the skin, as well as the peripheral circulatory system and lymph nodes. Cutaneous lesions related to ATL are polymorphous in appearance. Skin lesions are frequently observed in all the clinical subtypes. The prevalence of lesions reportedly ranges from 43% to 72% [21]. Furthermore, some reports have described patients who presented with cutaneous lesions only, remaining free for many years of leukemic changes or visceral invasion [22, 23]. Johno et al. [22] proposed a new category of ATL, cutaneous ATL (cATL), manifested throughout the entire course of disease by persistent skin lesions and which does not easily progress to leukemia or nodal lymphoma. Their findings also indicate that the prognosis of the tumoral type of ATL (MST: 26 months) is worse than that of the erythematopapular type (80 months) [22].

We previously investigated the HTLV-I proviral status and clinicopathological features of the cutaneous lesions of 80 cases with serum anti-ATL antibody (ATLA) to evaluate the relationship between the macroscopic/histopathological findings of the patients and patient outcome [23]. The MST of patients with the provirus was found to be 14 months, which was markedly shorter than the MST of patients negative for integrated proviral DNA (72 months). Of 46 cases with

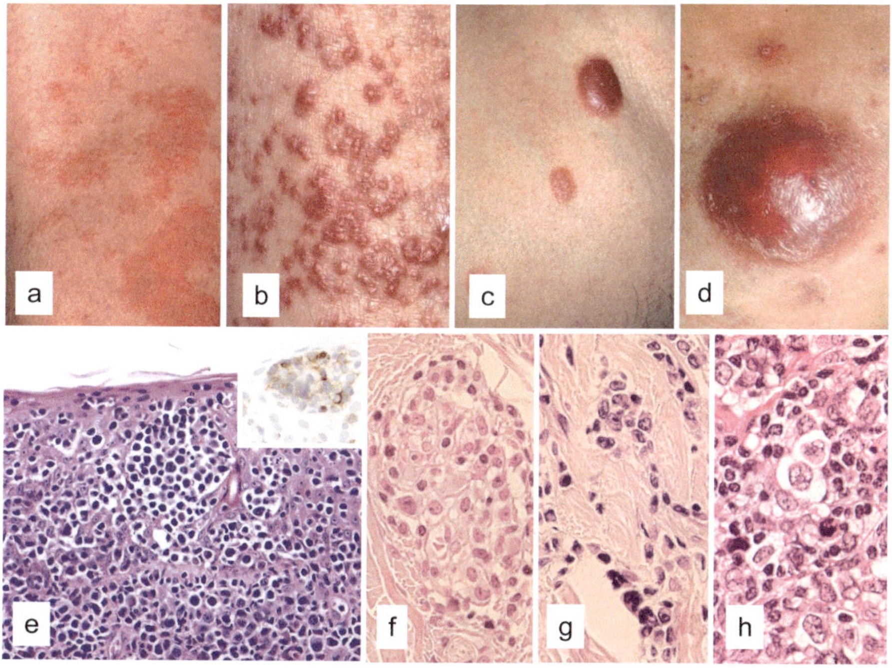


**Fig. 4.5** Macroscopic/histopathological findings of skin. (**a**) The macroscopic findings have been classified as erythema (**a**), papules (**b**), nodules (**c**), and tumor (**d**). Histopathological findings. The lymphoma cells have infiltrated the epidermis, producing Pautrier-like microabscesses. The lymphoma cells react with CD3 antibody (*inset*) (**e**). The lymphoma cell sizes are varied to small (**f**), medium sized (**g**), and large (**h**)

proviral DNA, 21 had solitary or multiple red nodules (including 3 with subcutaneous induration), 8 had multiple red papules, and 17 had erythema (Fig. 4.5). Patients with papules and tumors tended to have worse outcomes than those with erythema (Fig. 4.6).

Histopathological examination of the biopsy tissue from the erythematous lesions of the cases found perivascular or diffuse infiltration in the upper dermis by small- to medium-sized atypical lymphoid cells with mild to moderate nuclear atypia (Fig. 4.5). Mitotic figures were few in number. These atypical lymphoid cells had the phenotypes of peripheral T cells (CD1-, CD2+, CD3+, 45RO+, and usually CD4+) [21–23].

Histopathological examination of the biopsy tissue from nodular lesions of cases with nodules found infiltration by medium- to large-sized atypical lymphoid cells with round or irregular nuclei and small nucleoli. Mitotic figures were occasionally encountered. Biopsy tissue with a diffuse infiltration pattern also manifested atypical medium- to large-sized lymphoid cells. The outcome of patients with nodular or diffuse infiltration by medium- to large-sized lymphoma cells was worse than the

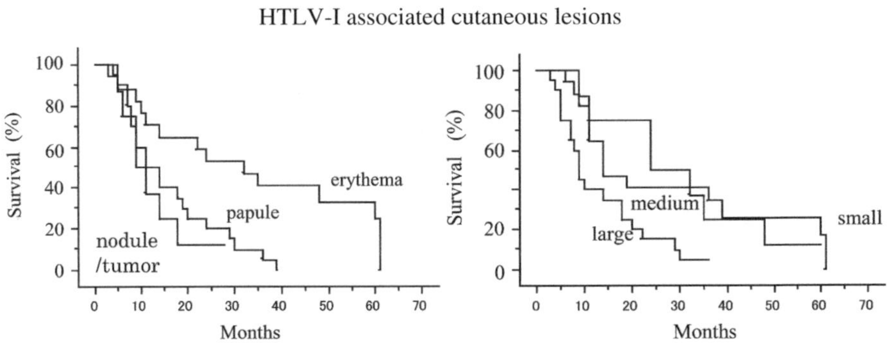


**Fig. 4.6** Survival of cutaneous lesions. Patients with papules, nodules, and tumors have poorer prognosis than those with erythema. The large-cell type have poorer prognosis than small and medium-sized type (Adapted from Ref. [23])

outcome of those with perivascular infiltration by small- to medium-sized lymphoma cells (Figs. 4.5 and 4.6) [23].

The macroscopic findings were fairly similar to the histopathological findings. The nodular lesions of cases with nodules showed nodular infiltration. The papular lesions showed nodular or diffuse infiltration. The erythematous lesions showed diffuse or perivascular infiltration. In this series of 80 cases, patients with nodules and papules had a worse outcome than those with erythema, and the histopathological analysis found that patients with nodular infiltration by atypical lymphoid cells had the worst outcome (MST: 9 months). The outcome of patients with diffusely infiltrated lesions (MST: 20 months) was somewhat better than the outcome of patients with perivascular infiltration of their lesions (MST: 24 months) [23].

### 4.1.5 Gastrointestinal Tract

The results of a few studies have suggested that HTLV-I may also be involved in the development of gastrointestinal T-cell lymphoma (GTL) [24, 25]. Sakata et al. [25] reported that 23–78% of ATL cases showed stomach invasion, and almost all of these patients were in an advanced clinical stage of the disease. While these findings indicate that gastric invasion by ATL cells occurs frequently during the advanced stage of ATL, there have also been reports of a few early-stage ATL cases with HTLV-I-associated GTL.

We analyzed 15 patients with HTLV-I-associated GTL [26]. The gastric lesions were located in the upper or middle corpus in eight cases and widely distributed in seven. Macroscopic examinations found ulcerated masses, erosions, or tumors. Histopathological examination found three types of lesions. One type showed diffuse infiltration by atypical medium-sized lymphoid cells with round or irregular

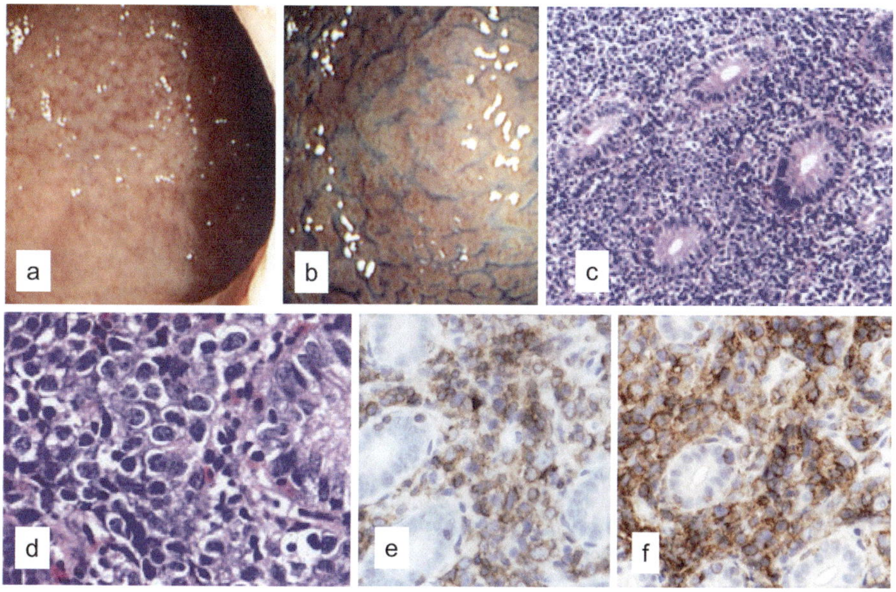


**Fig. 4.7** Macroscopic/histopathological findings of gastrointestinal tracts. (**a**) Endoscopy demonstrated edematous and reddish mucosa in large intestine. (**b**) The spreading methylene blue on the mucosa surface enabled to discriminate the lesions. (**c**) The large intestine shows a diffuse infiltration of lymphoma cells in the mucosa. (**d**) The lymphoma cells are pleomorphic medium-sized and large-cell type. The lymphoma cells react with CD3 (**e**) and CD4 (**f**) antibody

nuclei. A second type showed diffuse infiltration by medium- and large-sized pleomorphic lymphoid cells with round or irregular nuclei. The third type, which occurred in rare cases, had diffuse proliferation of large to giant anaplastic cells with round or lobulated nuclei, distinct nucleoli, and abundant cytoplasm. Cohesive growth patterns were detected (Figs. 4.7 and 4.8). Among all three types, the destruction of gastric glands by infiltrating lymphoma cells was obvious. These patients all had poor outcomes, dying within 2 years of treatment. Four cases in this series showed no evidence of leukemic changes, but nine cases showed atypical lymphoid cells in the peripheral blood (1–2% of lymphocytes were atypical) [26]. Rare cases showed small and large intestinal lesions, which appeared on endoscopy as multiple ulcers or erosive changes [24].

### 4.1.6 *Liver*

ATL involvement of the liver is mainly seen in the portal area, which shows infiltration by atypical medium- to large-sized lymphoid cells with irregular nuclei. Destruction of the limiting plate of hepatocytes is occasionally seen, and in some

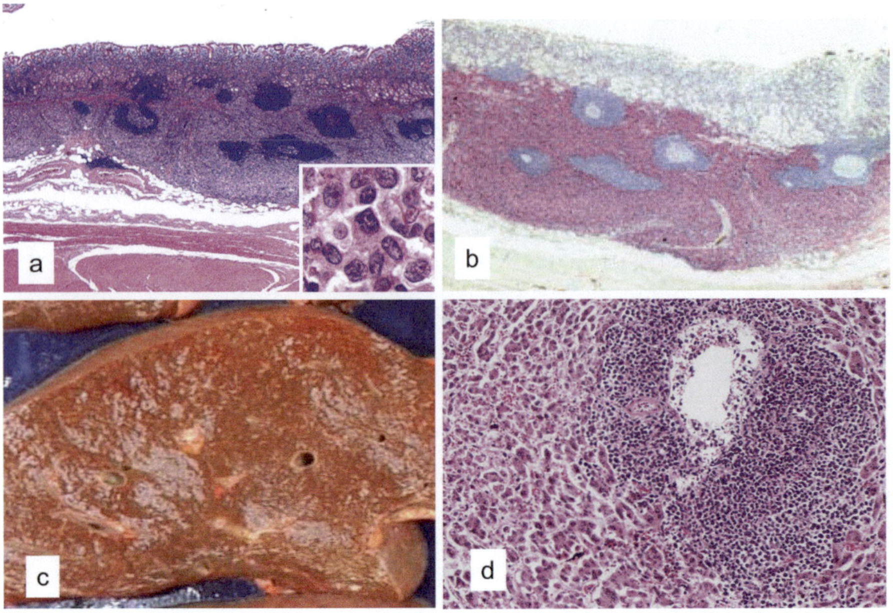


**Fig. 4.8** Histological findings of stomach and liver. (**a**) The stomach shows a tumorous lesion with a diffuse proliferation of lymphoma cells with anaplastic large-cell features (inset). (**b**) The lymphoma cells react with CD3. (**c**) The liver shows diffuse swelling but no local lesions. (**d**) The portal area of the liver shows a diffuse infiltration of atypical lymphoid cells

cases, there is sinus infiltration. Fibrosis is rare (Fig. 4.8c, d). Mitotic features are occasionally encountered. [14]

### *4.1.7 Bone Marrow*

ATL involvement of the bone marrow is occasionally seen, even in cases with a leukemic blood picture, as are patchy infiltrates of atypical lymphoid cells with irregular or round nuclei in the marrow cavity, sometimes near bone trabeculae. Clinically, hypercalcemia is an important laboratory finding associated with ATL. Absorption of bone accompanied by periosteal fibrosis, such as seen in osteitis fibrosa generalisata, may or may not be accompanied by tumor cell infiltrates (Fig. 4.9). Increased numbers of osteoclasts are sometimes seen in the peritrabecular spaces (Fig. 4.9) [14].

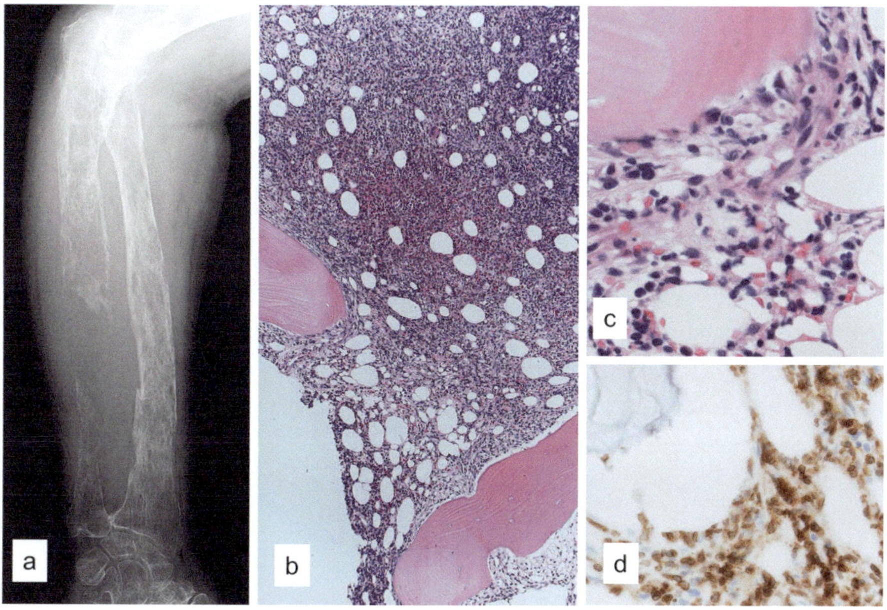


**Fig. 4.9** Bone and bone marrow of ATL. (**a**) A radiograph of the leg shows extensive lytic bone lesions. (**b**) The bone marrow shows diffuse infiltration of lymphoma cells. (**c**) The lymphoma cells are pleomorphic medium-sized and large-cell type. And osteoclasts of the peri-trabeculae are increased in number. (**d**) The lymphoma cells react with CD3 antibody

## 4.2 Nonneoplastic Lesions

### *4.2.1 HTLV-I-Associated Myelopathy/Tropical Spastic Paraparesis (HAM/TSP)*

The first symptoms are weakness of the lower limbs and lumbar pain, although the initial complaint can be sensory in nature, such as tingling, burning, or pins and needles. Urinary and sexual problems can also be initial symptoms [27].

The disease mainly affects the spinal cord, particularly the lateral and anterior columns, where bilateral loss of myelin and axons has been observed, mainly along the neural tract. Perivascular and parenchymal infiltration by lymphocytes and macrophages, as well as astrocytosis, have been found in the white and gray matter of the spinal cord, while blood vessels in the spinal cord and in the subarachnoid space of the spinal cord have shown hyaline thickening of the media and adventitia, associated with infiltrating lymphocytes (Fig. 4.10a). The lymphocytes have not shown nuclear atypia, and mitotic figures have rarely been encountered. The spinal lesion is associated with dense perivascular mononuclear cell infiltrates, largely CD8+ lymphocytes [28].

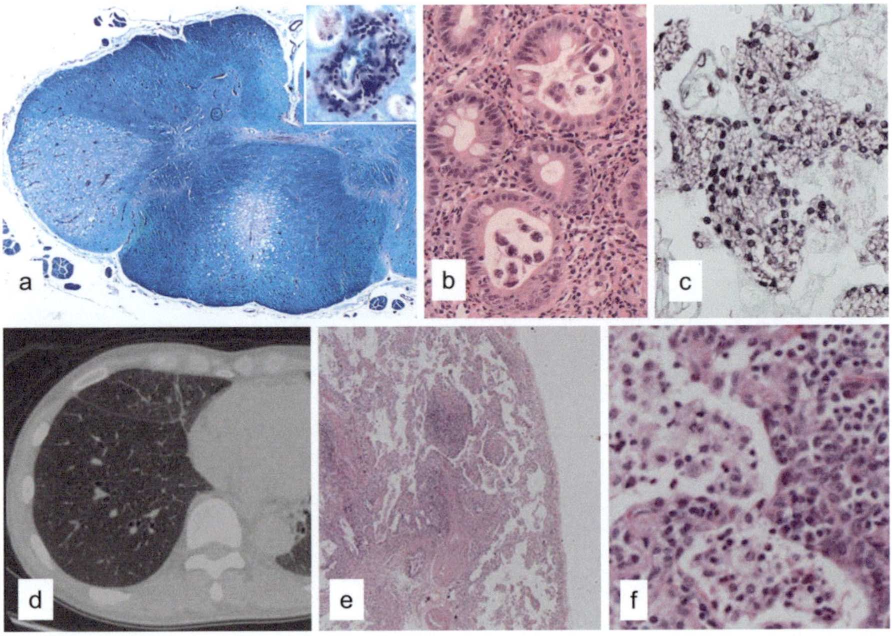


**Fig. 4.10** Histology of HAM and immunodeficient disorders. (**a**) HAM mainly affects the spinal cord, particularly the lateral and anterior columns, where loss of myelin and axon, accompanied by dense lymphocytic perivascular infiltration (inset) (Kluver-Barrera staining). (**b**) Strongyloides stercoralis was detected in the gastric glands. (**c**) Pneumocystis carinii was identified in the alveolar spaces by means of Grocott staining. (**d**) HTLV-I-associated bronchopneumopathy (HAB) displays diffuse reticular shadow in CT. (**e**) The histology shows a proliferation of bronchial mucosa epithelium with an infiltration of lymphocytes. (**f**) The lymphocytes show no nuclear atypia

### *4.2.2 HTLV-I-Associated Uveitis (HAU)*

Based on seroepidemiological, clinical, and virological data, it can be concluded that HTLV-I is closely associated with a certain type of uveitis. Uveitis is a vision-threatening inflammatory disorder affecting the intraocular tissues (iris, ciliary body, vitreous body, optic nerve, retina, choroid). Histopathological examination has found that the intraocular tissues are infiltrated by a number of inflammatory cells, including lymphocytes and histiocytes. The lesion is characterized by a granulomatous or nongranulomatous reaction accompanied by vitreous opacity and retinal vasculitis. The lymphocytes do not show nuclear atypia, and mitotic figures are rarely encountered. [29]

### 4.2.3 *HTLV-I-Associated Bronchopneumopathy or Diffuse Panbronchiolitis (HAB)*

Kimura et al. [30] reported that some individuals with idiopathic interstitial pneumonia and diffuse panbronchiolitis possessed an anti-ATL antibody (ATLA). They postulated an association between HTLV-I infection and idiopathic interstitial pneumonia and diffuse panbronchiolitis.

Histopathologically, there is a proliferation of bronchial epithelial mucosa accompanied by thickening of the basement membrane and an infiltrate in the epithelial layer and mucosa propria, predominantly consisting of lymphocytes together with some plasma cells, histiocytes, and neutrophils (Fig. 4.10d–f). The lymphocytes are usually small; and nuclear atypia and mitotic features are rare, while in the alveolar areas there is mild fibrosis and edema of the alveolar wall and infiltration by lymphocytes and some plasma cells.

In cases with leukemia/lymphoma invasion, however, there is prominent diffuse infiltration by atypical lymphocytes with irregular nuclei. Nodular proliferation is also present in these cases.

### 4.2.4 *Opportunistic Infections*

Opportunistic infections occur frequently in patients with ATL [4]. In addition, HTLV-I-infected carriers seem to have an increased risk of strongyloidiasis, which suggests a possible subclinical immunodeficiency. HTLV-I-infected individuals from areas where *Strongyloides stercoralis* is highly endemic should probably have regular fecal examinations (Fig. 4.10b, c). Other reported infections associated with HTLV-I carriers include crusted scabies, disseminated molluscum contagiosum, and extrapulmonary histoplasmosis [4].

## References

1. Takatsuki K. Overview of adult T-cell leukemia/lymphoma. Jpn Soc Res. 1985;25:97–103.
2. Poiesz BJ, Ruscetti FW, Mier JW, et al. T-cell lines established from human T-lymphocytic neoplasias by direct response to T-cell growth factor. Proc Natl Acad Sci U S A. 1980;77:6815–9.
3. Gonçalves DU, Proietti FA, Ribas JG, Araújo MG, Pinheiro SR, Guedes AC, Carneiro-Proietti AB. Epidemiology, treatment, and prevention of human T-cell leukemia.Virus type 1-associated diseases. Clin Microbiol Rev. 2010;23(3):577–89.
4. Takatsuki K, Yamaguchi K, Watanabe T, Mochizuki M. Adult T-cell leukemia and HTLV-1 related disease. Gann Mono Can Res. 1992;32:1–15.
5. Osame M, Usuku K, Izumo S, et al. HTLV-I associated myeopathy, a new clinical entity. Lancet. 1986;i:1013–4.

6. Gessain A, Barin F, Vernat JC, et al. Antibodies to human T-lymphotropic virus type-I in patients with tropical spastic paraparesis. Lancet. 1985;ii:407–9.
7. Whittaker SJ, Ng YL, Rustin M, Levene G, McGibbon DH, Smith NP. HTLV-1-associated cutaneous disease: a clinicopathological and molecular study of patients from the UK. Br J Dermatol. 1993;128(5):483–92.
8. Blayney DW, Jaffe ES, Blattner WA, Cossman J, Robert-Guroff M, Longo DL, Bunn Jr PA, Gallo RC. The human T-cell leukemia/lymphoma virus associated with American adult T-cell leukemia/lymphoma. Blood. 1983;62(2):401–5.
9. Shimoyama M. Diagnostic criteria and classification of clinical subtypes of adult T-cell leukaemia-lymphoma: a report from the Lymphoma Study Group (1984-87). Br J Haematol. 1991;79(3):428–37.
10. Tsukasaki K, Hermine O, Bazarbachi A, Ratner L, Ramos JC, Harrington Jr W, O'Mahony D, Janik JE, Bittencourt AL, Taylor GP, Yamaguchi K, Utsunomiya A, Tobinai K, Watanabe T. Definition, prognostic factors, treatment, and response criteria of adult T-cell leukemia-lymphoma: a proposal from an international consensus meeting. J Clin Oncol. 2009;27 (3):453–9.
11. Ohshima K, Kikuchi M, Yoshida T, Masuda Y, Kimura N. Lymph nodes in incipient adult T-cell leukemia lymphoma with Hodgkin's disease-like histologic features. Cancer. 1991;67:1622–8.
12. Ohshima K, Kikuchi M, Masuda Y, et al. HTLV-I associated lymphadenitis. Cancer. 1992;69:239–48.
13. Ohshima K, Suzumiya J, Sato M, et al. Survival of patients with HTLV-I-associated lymph node lesions. J Pathol. 1999;189:539–45.
14. Kikuchi M, Takeshita M, Ohshima K, Yoshida T. Pathology of adult T-cell leukemia/lymphoma and HTLV-I associated organopathies. Gann Mono Can Res. 1992;39:69–80.
15. Takeshita M, Ohshima K, Akamatsu M, et al. CD30-positive anaplastic large cell lymphoma in a human T-cell lymphotrophic virus-I endemic area. Hum Pathol. 1995;26:614–9.
16. Karube K, Suzumiya J, Okamoto M, et al. Adult T cell lymphoma/leukemia with angioimmunoblastic T cell lymphoma-like features: report of 11 cases. Am J Surg Pathol. 2007;31:216–23.
17. Ohshima K. Pathological features of diseases associated with human T-cell leukemia virus type I. Cancer Sci. 2007;98(6):772–8.
18. Karube K, Ohshima K, Tsuchiya T, Yamaguchi T, Kawano R, Suzumiya J, Utsunomiya A, Harada M, Kikuchi M. Expression of FoxP3, a key molecule in CD4CD25 regulatory T cells, in adult T-cell leukaemia/lymphoma cells. Br J Haematol. 2004;126(1):81–4.
19. Tsukasaki K, Tsushima H, Yamamura M, Hata T, Murata K, Maeda T, Atogami S, Sohda H, Momita S, Ideda S, Katamine S, Yamada Y, Kamihira S, Tomonaga M. Integration patterns of HTLV-I provirus in relation to the clinical course of ATL: frequent clonal change at crisis from indolent disease. Blood. 1997;89(3):948–56.
20. Ohshima K, Suzumiya J, Kato A, et al. Clonal HTLV-I-infected CD4+ lymphocytes and non-clonal non-HTLV-I-infected giant cells in incipient ATLL with Hodgkin-like histologic features. Int J Cancer. 1997;72:592–8.
21. Dosaka N, Tanaka T, Miyachi Y, et al. Examination of HTLV-1 integration in the skin lesions of various type of adult T-cell leukemia (ATL): independence of cutaneous-type ATL confirmed by Southern blot analysis. J Invest Dermatol. 1991;96:196–200.
22. Johno M, Ohishi M, Kojo Y, et al. Cutaneous manifestations of adult T cell leukemia/ lymphoma. In: Takatsuki K, Hinuma Y, Yoshida M, editors. Advances in adult T-cell leukemia and HTLV-1 research. Tokyo: Japan Scientific Society Press; 1992. p. 33–41.
23. Yamaguchi T, Ohshima K, Karube K, et al. Clinicopathological features of cutaneous lesions of adult T-cell leukemia/lymphoma. Br J Dermatol. 2005;152:76–81.
24. Utsunomiya A, Hanada S. (1990) Clinical and pathological features of gastrointestinal lesions in patients with adult T cell leukemia. J Clin Exp Hematol 30, 31–48 (Japanese).

25. Sakata H, Kazuma F. (1997) Adult T-cell leukemia and gastric lesion. G.I. Res 5; 4–7 (Japanese).
26. Hatano B, Ohshima K, Katoh A, et al. Non-HTLV-1-associated primary gastric T-cell lymphomas show cytotoxic activity: clinicopathological, immunohistochemical characteristics and TIA-1 expression in 31 cases. Histopathology. 2002;41:421–36.
27. Orland JR, Engstrom J, Fridey J, Sacher RA, Smith JW, Nass C, Garratty G, Newman B, Smith D, Wang B, Loughlin K, Murphy EL. HTLV outcomes study. Prevalence and clinical features of HTLV neurologic disease in the HTLV outcomes study. Neurology. 2003;61 (11):1588–94.
28. Bangham CRM, Osame M. Cellular immune response to HTLV-1. Oncogene. 2005;24 (39):6035–46.
29. Mochizuki M, Watanabe T, Yamaguchi K, Yoshimura K, Nakashima S, Shirao M, Araki S, Takatsuki K, Mori S, Miyata N. Uveitis associated with human T-cell lymphotropic virus type I. Am J Ophthalmol. 1992;114(2):123–9.
30. Kimura I. (1992) HABA (HTLV-I associated bronchiolo-alveolar disorder). Nihon Kyobu Shikkan Gakkai Zasshi 30(5):787–795 (Japanese).

# Chapter 5
# Immunophenotype

**Kaoru Uchimaru**

## 5.1 Typical Immunophenotype of Adult T-cell leukemia/lymphoma (ATL) Cells

Adult T-cell leukemia/lymphoma (ATL) is a malignancy of CD4(+) peripheral T cells. Accordingly, ATL cells express T cell-associated antigens (pan-T markers) such as CD2, CD3, and CD5 but usually lack CD7 [1]. Most ATL cells express CD45RO, which is expressed on effector/memory T cells, and not the naïve T cell marker CD45RA. Because at least one of these pan-T markers, particularly CD5 and/or CD7, is usually lost in T cell malignancies [2] and CD7 is also lost on tumor cells in most cases with Sezary Syndrome or mycosis fungoides [3], loss of CD7 is not specific for ATL. ATL cells usually express CD4 but not CD8 antigen. However, in some cases, the tumor cells express CD8. In these cases, some express CD4 and others do not. The incidence of the typical CD4(+)/CD8(−) phenotype in ATL cases is around 80% and 10–20% of the cases are CD8(+), that is, CD4(−)/CD8(+) or double-positive [4]. There are also CD4/CD8 double-negative cases. The CD8 antigen is composed of α and β subunits and the CD8αα homodimer can be induced on the surface of CD4 T cells [5]. ATL cells can reversibly express CD4 and CD8α antigen and sometimes CD8β antigen [6, 7]. Yamada and colleagues [7] reported the induction of a CD8αα(+) cell line from CD4(+) ATL cells. Most CD8(+) ATL cases express CD8αα homodimer on the surface of tumor cells. These results suggest that most CD8(+) ATL cells are derived from CD4(+) cells.

ATL cells express CD25, which is the α chain of the IL-2 receptor. It is expressed on activated T cells and B cells [8, 9]. Furthermore, most resting memory T cells express CD25 [10], and it is one of the most important markers of regulatory T cells

K. Uchimaru (✉)
Department of Hematology/Oncology, Research Hospital, Institute of Medical Science, the University of Tokyo, Tokyo, Japan
e-mail: uchimaru@ims.u-tokyo.ac.jp



T. Watanabe, T. Fukushima (eds.), *Adult T-cell Leukemia/Lymphoma*,
DOI 10.1007/978-4-431-56523-9_5

[11]. So, though it is also a well-known Tac antigen expressed on ATL cells [12], it is not a specific marker of ATL. Indeed, presently, there is no known single surface marker that can be used to discriminate between ATL cells and other T cell malignancies.

CD25 has been a therapeutic target for ATL. Denileukin diftitox is a fusion protein of the diphtheria toxin and the receptor-binding domain of IL-2, which can bind to CD25 [13, 14]. It is active for cutaneous T-cell lymphoma and peripheral T-cell lymphoma (PTCL) and may be active for ATL.

Recently, a phase I/II clinical trial of the monoclonal anti-CD25 antibody daclizumab was conducted for aggressive and indolent ATL. Some chronic and smoldering ATL patients achieved partial remission, but it failed to show activity against aggressive ATL [15]. LMB-2 is an anti-CD25 antibody Fv fragment fused to a pseudomonas exotoxin [16]. Promising results were reported in a phase II clinical trial of LMB-2 combined with cyclophosphamide and fludarabine [17].

Typical ATL cells are morphologically distinct. They have a multi-lobulated nucleus and basophilic cytoplasm and have been called "flower cells," but the morphology of ATL cells is diverse and it is often difficult to morphologically distinguish ATL cells from non-ATL cells, particularly in indolent-type ATL cases. In acute myeloid/lymphoblastic leukemia, leukemic cells can be clearly detected as CD45-diminished cells using fluorescence-activated cell sorting (FACS) analysis. For ATL, there is not yet a widely accepted FACS system that can detect tumor cells. As described above, typical ATL cells express CD3 and most cases lack CD7 expression. In a previous study, CD3 expression decreased after Human T-Cell Leukemia Virus Type 1 (HTLV-1) infection, correlating with the downregulation of CD7 expression [18–20]. Using these data, another study constructed a multi-color flow cytometric analysis system to discriminate acute-type ATL cells from non-ATL cells [21]. In this FACS system, ATL cells are detected as a CD3-dim/CD7(−) population within the CD4(+) population, in which monocytes are gated out according to CD14 expression. Representative data are shown in Fig. 5.1. ATL cells are detected as a CD3-dim/CD7(−) population with high purity. Flow cytometric analysis of ATL cells in the peripheral blood is useful for an accurate estimation of the efficacy of treatment.

## 5.2 Chemokine Receptor

Chemokines are cytokines that induce chemotaxis and the activation of leukocytes. Chemokines bind to their specific receptors: 18 chemokine receptors have been identified [22]. Chemokines and their receptor systems are important in lymphocyte differentiation and migration. T lymphocytes are divided into various subsets according to their function and these functions depend on their chemokine receptor expression [23]. Among them, CCR4 is expressed selectively on Th2 cells and regulatory T cells [24, 25]. CCR4 is a characteristic marker of ATL cells. In one study, 88.3% of ATL cases expressed CCR4 but only 4.9% expressed CXCR3, a typical marker of Th1 cells [26]. In addition, compared to CCR4(−) ATL patients,

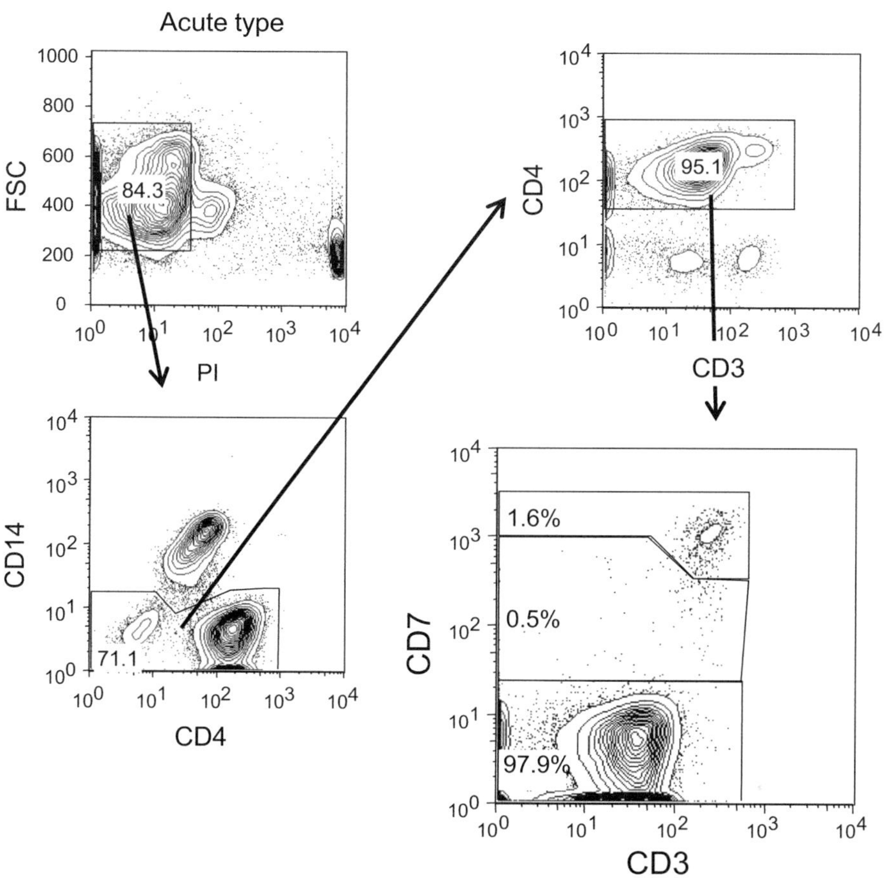


**Fig. 5.1** CD3/7 plot of ATL cells

CCR4(+) ATL patients were significantly more likely to have skin involvement because cutaneous endothelia expressed the CCR4 ligand thymus and activation-regulated cytokine (TARC) and had significantly worse prognoses. The authors reported that CCR4 expression was an independent and significant prognostic factor of aggressive ATL.

Peripheral T cell lymphoma not otherwise specified (PTCL-NOS) is a heterogeneous clinical entity, and various chemokine receptors are expressed on the tumor cells. From the viewpoint of chemokine receptor expression patterns, PTCL-NOS can be classified into three groups: the CCR4, CCR3, and CXCR3 types. In gene expression profile analyses using DNA tip chips arrays, ATL, angioimmunoblastic T cell lymphoma (AILT), and anaplastic large cell lymphoma (ALCL) had tendencies to cluster, whereas some PTCL-NOS cases clustered with ATL, some with AILT, and others with ALCL. They expressed CCR4, CXCR3, and CCR3, respectively. Furthermore, an array comparative genomic hybridization (array CGH) study revealed that a pattern of genomic imbalance in CCR4-positive

PTCL-NOS was very close to that of lymphoma-type ATL. The subgroup had similar prognoses to ATL, AILT, and ALCL, respectively [27]. These data may suggest that CCR4-positive PTCL-NOS, regardless of HTLV-1 infection, may share some common oncogenic pathways with ATL, particularly in the lymphoma type [27].

CCR4 may be a therapeutic molecular target, and an anti-CCR4 antibody has been developed to treat CCR4-positive lymphoid malignancies. Mogamulizumab is a defucosylated humanized anti-CCR4 antibody [28]. In a phase II study conducted in Japan, mogamulizumab achieved an overall response rate of 50% for refractory or relapsed ATL patients, and 30.8% showed complete remission [29]. Recently, a multicenter, randomized phase II study that compared combination chemotherapy (mLSG15) with or without mogamulizumab reported that adding mogamulizumab to mLSG15 increased the overall response rate and the proportion of patients who had complete remission [30]. As CCR4 is also a marker for regulatory T cells, mogamulizumab also depletes regulatory T cells (Tregs; see Sect. 5.3). This may contribute to enhanced anti-tumor immunity, but it may also exaggerate graft-versus-host disease after allogeneic hematopoietic stem cell transplantation, and should be carefully revealed whether mogamulizumab can be used safely before allogeneic stem cell transplantation in the future.

Surveillance studies on chemokine expression other than CCR4 have revealed that ATL cells express CCR1, CCR7, CCR8, CCR10, and CXCR4 but barely express CCR2, CCR3, CCR5, CCR6, CCR9, CXCR1, CXCR2, CXCR3, or CXCR5 [31–33]. Because chemokines are important for chemotaxis and tissue-homing of T cells, these chemokine expression profiles have a significant influence on ATL cell biology. As mentioned above, CCR4 is a receptor for TARC (CCL17) and macrophage-derived chemokine (MDC, CCL22). Skin keratinocytes, dendritic cells, and endothelial cells produce CCL17 and CCL22, and thus CCR4 expression is likely one reason why ATL cells infiltrate skin lesions [34]. Moreover, considering that CCL27 (cutaneous T-cell attracting chemokine; CTACK) is the ligand for CCL10 produced by epidermal keratinocytes, CCR10 expression may contribute to skin infiltration of ATL cells. Another CCR10 ligand, CCL28 (mucosa-associated epithelial chemokine; MEK), has been reported to be expressed in the intestinal mucosa [35, 36]; thus, CCR10 expression may explain the frequent gastrointestinal infiltration in ATL [33].

## 5.3 Regulatory T Cell Markers

Tregs are a distinct subset of T cells that suppress aberrant or excessive immune responses, maintaining self-tolerance [37]. Tregs express CD4 and CD25, which they share with Th2 cells and ATL cells. Furthermore, they express CCR4 and CCR8 chemokine receptors, which are also typically expressed on ATL cells. Given these immunophenotypical similarities between Tregs and ATL cells and the strong immunosuppressive activity of ATL cells [7], expression of regulatory

T cell-associated molecules on ATL cells has been extensively surveyed. Glucocorticoid-induced tumor necrosis factor receptor-related protein (GITR, CD357) and cytotoxic T-lymphocyte-associated protein 4 (CTLA4, CD152) have been reported to be key markers of functional Tregs [38, 39]. GITR is a member of the TNF receptor superfamily and is mainly expressed in lymphoid tissues, including Treg cells. CTLA4 has been reported to be a costimulatory molecule of Tregs. Markedly higher expression of GITR has been reported in primary ATL cells [40]. Regarding CTLA4, CD4(+)CD25(+) cells in the peripheral blood express considerable levels of CTLA4 in representative ATL cases [41]. These data, along with the immunosuppressive activity of ATL cells, suggest that ATL cells may originate from Tregs.

FoxP3 is a transcription factor that is essential for Treg function [42]. It is a master regulator of Treg development and function. Several studies have revealed that ATL cells express FoxP3 [40, 43] and these findings further suggest that ATL cells may be derived from Treg cells. In the peripheral blood of HTLV-1 asymptomatic carriers, HTLV-1 is frequently detected in CD4(+)FoxP3(+) cells [44]. One possible explanation for FoxP3 expression on HTLV-1-infected CD4(+) T cells is induction by HTLV-1 basic leucine zipper factor (HBZ). HBZ is encoded on the minus strand of the HTLV-1 provirus [45] and is constitutively expressed from the 3′-LTR. HBZ transgenic mice develop T-cell lymphomas that express CD4, indicating that HBZ has transforming activity for T cells [46]. Tumor cells of transgenic mice resemble ATL cells and cells infected with HTLV-1 in HTLV-1 asymptomatic carriers. These lymphoma cells express FoxP3, and HBZ directly induces FoxP3 expression in CD4(+) T cells. These results indicate that FoxP3 expression can be induced by HBZ in cells infected with HTLV-1 and as FoxP3 is a master regulator of the Treg phenotype, cells infected with HTLV-1 may exhibit a Treg-like phenotype. It may be that ATL cells do not necessarily originate from Treg cells and the origin of ATL cells should be determined in future studies.

## 5.4 Transferrin Receptor

The transferrin receptor (CD71) is a glycoprotein that plays a key role in the regulation of iron metabolism and cell growth [47, 48]. It is expressed constitutively on actively proliferating cells, such as hematopoietic cells and enterocytes of the intestinal mucosa [49]. HTLV-1 infection upregulates surface transferrin receptor expression by changing its distribution between the cytoplasm and cell membrane [50]. In ATL patients, tumor cells have been reported to express high levels of this receptor, particularly in acute-type ATL patients [51]. Its expression in indolent-type ATL is lower than in aggressive-type ATL. Blockade of the transferrin receptor using a monoclonal antibody suppresses the proliferation of cells infected with HTLV-1. An anti-transferrin receptor antibody can block the binding of transferrin to the transferrin receptor and inhibit cell proliferation and induce apoptosis [51]. These data suggest that a monoclonal antibody for the transferrin

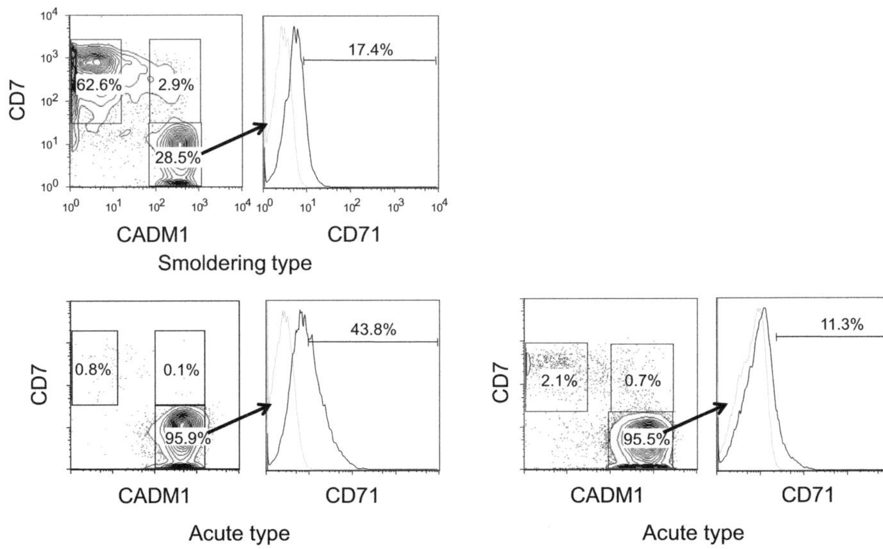


**Fig. 5.2** Transferrin receptor expression on ATL cells

receptor may represent a novel immunotherapy for ATL. Clinical assessments of anti-transferrin receptor monoclonal antibodies for ATL treatment have been undertaken. The expression level of the receptor may be variable even in aggressive ATL cells (Fig. 5.2, lower right) and should be determined in each case.

The transferrin receptor is relevant to cell proliferation and there is a possibility that a non-proliferating fraction does not express it. Yamaguchi et al. [52] investigated cancer stem cells in a Tax-transgenic mouse model of ATL and identified putative cancer stem cells in a side population that showed the immunophenotype of CD38(−), CD71(−), and CD117(+). These results suggest that there may be a tumor cell population that does not express the transferrin receptor in ATL patients. The distribution of its expression in cells infected with HTLV-1 and ATL cells should be investigated further.

## 5.5 Death Receptors

The Fas receptor, also called CD95, is a transmembrane glycoprotein belonging to the tumor necrosis factor (TNF) receptor family [53]. Fas induces apoptosis by binding to Fas ligand (FasL) and is important in the regulation of physiological and pathological cell death. Receptors that induce cell death are called death receptors and Fas is a representative death receptor, along with the TNF-related apoptosis-inducing ligand (TRAIL) receptor. Regulation of cell proliferation and cell death is crucial in physiological states, and deregulation of apoptosis can induce clonal expansion, leading to malignancy. In ATL cells, Fas expression is paradoxically upregulated. Among ATL subtypes, chronic-type ATL cells express significantly higher levels of Fas than acute-type ATL cells [54]. Despite high expression of Fas, ATL cells are resistant to FasL-induced apoptosis. Several mechanisms, such as induction of cellular FADD-like IL-1β converting enzyme (FLICE) inhibitory protein (c-FLIP) by Tax [55–57] and expression of truncated Fas, which deletes the transmembrane domain and suppresses membrane-bound Fas signals in a dominant negative manner [58, 59], confer this resistance in ATL cells. c-FLIP profoundly inhibits Fas-mediated apoptosis by preventing the formation of death-inducing signaling complex (DISC) [56, 60]. TRAIL belongs to the TNF gene superfamily, which induces apoptosis in various tumor cells [61]. The TRAIL receptor has four isoforms, of which TRAIL R1 and R2 are the active forms, and most ATL cells express a TRAIL receptor, principally TRAIL R2 [62]. Despite expression of TRAIL R2, ATL cells are also resistant to TRAIL-induced cell death due to overexpression of c-FLIP [55, 56, 63].

## 5.6 CADM1

Tumor suppressor of lung cancer 1 (TSLC1) is a tumor suppressor gene identified in non-small cell lung cancer [64]. It is frequently inactivated in various cancers, such as esophageal, gastric, pancreatic, breast, and uterine cervical cancer [64]. It belongs to the immunoglobulin superfamily and is involved in the formation of epithelial structure. It has also been called immunoglobulin superfamily 4 (IGSF4), Necl-2, SgIGSF, RA175, and SynCAM1, depending on its observed function, but is now called cell adhesion molecule 1 (CADM1) [65, 66]. CADM1 is expressed in most tissues, except peripheral lymphocytes. In hematopoietic cells, it is weakly expressed in erythrocytes and more weakly in neutrophils and monocytes but is not expressed in T lymphocytes [67]. A fraction of CD4(+)CD25(+)FoxP3(+) Tregs in the peripheral blood of healthy volunteers express CADM1, but the expression level is low [68].

Although CADM1 was first identified as a tumor suppressor gene, ectopic high expression has been reported in ATL [69]. Morishita and colleagues examined gene expression profiles of more than 12,000 genes using microarrays in acute-type ATL cells and found that CADM1 was one of the three most upregulated genes and confirmed their expression in acute- and chronic-type ATL cells [67]. The same group further studied CD4(+)CADM1(+) cells in ATL patients and revealed that the proportion of CD4(+)CD25(+) double-positive cells and abnormal lymphocytes correlated well with that of CD4(+)CADM1(+) cells in the peripheral blood [68]. Furthermore, they showed that the proportion of CADM1(+) cells in CD4-positive cells in the peripheral blood of HTLV-1 asymptomatic carriers correlated well with the HTLV-1 DNA copy number [68, 69]. These results suggest that CADM1 may be a marker for cells infected with HTLV-1, even in the early phase of the oncogenic process in ATL development.

Kobayashi et al. [70] constructed a multi-color FACS analysis system using CADM1 and CD7 expression. Briefly, dead cells were initially excluded and monocytes were gated out as CD14(+)/CD4-dim cells on a CD4 versus CD14 plot. After CD4(+) T lymphocytes were gated on a CD3 versus CD4 plot, a CADM1 versus CD7 plot was prepared (Fig. 5.3). Representative data are shown in Fig. 5.4. Acute-type ATL cells were detected and highly purified as a CADM1(+) CD7-negative population (N, Fig. 5.4, top left). When analyzing indolent-type ATL cells, such as smoldering and chronic cells, two other populations can be clearly detected: CADM1(+)/CD7-dim and CADM1(−)/CD7(+) (P, D, Fig. 5.4, top, middle, and right). In asymptomatic carriers, these three populations can be detected and the proportions of the D and N populations increase as disease status progresses (Fig. 5.4, bottom, middle, and right). Clonally expanding cells can be detected in the D and N populations by inverse PCR (Fig. 5.5a, b) and major expanding clone (s) exist in advanced asymptomatic carriers and ATL patients. These D and N populations, detected in the peripheral blood of advanced asymptomatic carriers and indolent ATL patients, have some common properties with aggressive ATL cells, such as severe suppression of miR31 expression and aberrant splicing patterns of Ikaros family genes [70–73]. These results suggest that the immunophenotype of cells infected with HTLV-1 changed from CD7(+)CADM1(−), through CD7-dim/ CADM1(+), to CD7(−)/CADM1(+). The CD7(+)/CADM1-negative population

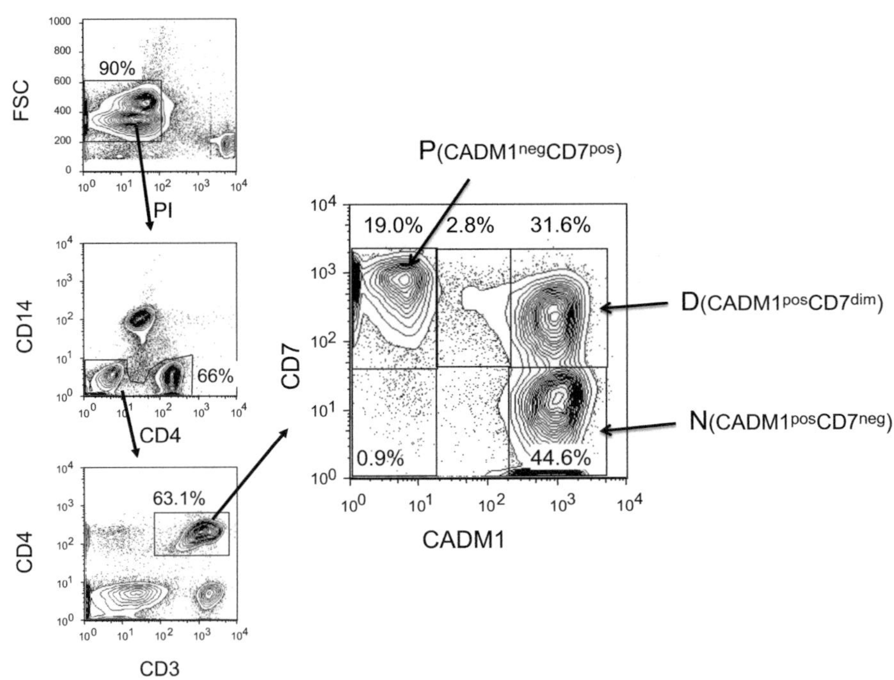


**Fig. 5.3** CADM1/CD7 plot of ATL cells (HAS-2G)

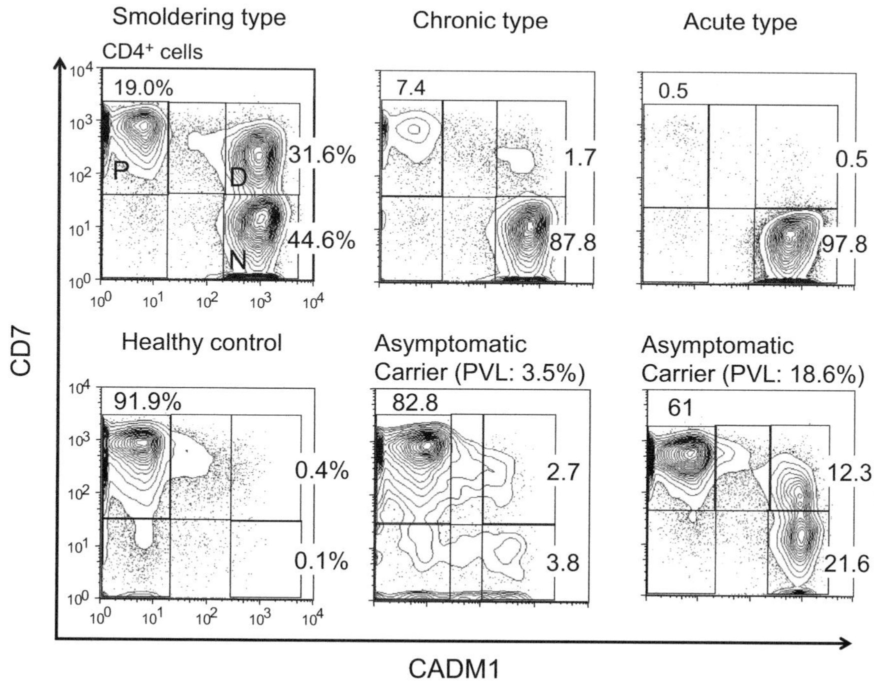


**Fig. 5.4** Representative CADM1/CD7 plot of various states of cells infected with HTLV-1

includes some cells infected with HTLV-1 which can be detected by real-time PCR, so there are some CADM1-negative cells infected with HTLV-1, although most HTLV-1 cells are CADM1(+), particularly in advanced asymptomatic carriers and ATL patients [70]. This multi-color FACS system using CD7 and CADM1 was named the second-generation HTLV-1 analysis system (HAS-2G) and is useful for monitoring patients infected with HTLV-1 and promising for detecting high-risk carriers for ATL development [74]. Cell sorting using HAS-2G makes it possible to separate and purify an intermediate-state population of cells infected with HTLV-1 that will develop into ATL and be useful for analyzing the oncogenic process to ATL.

## 5.7 CD26

CD26 is a glycoprotein that possesses dipeptidyl peptidase IV (DPPIV) activity in its extracellular domain. It is expressed in various tissues, including the kidney, lung, liver, melanocytes, and T cells [75]. CD26 is a multifunctional protein whose functions include T cell co-stimulation and immune regulation [76]. Changes in CD26 expression have been reported in lymphoid malignancy. Tumor cells of

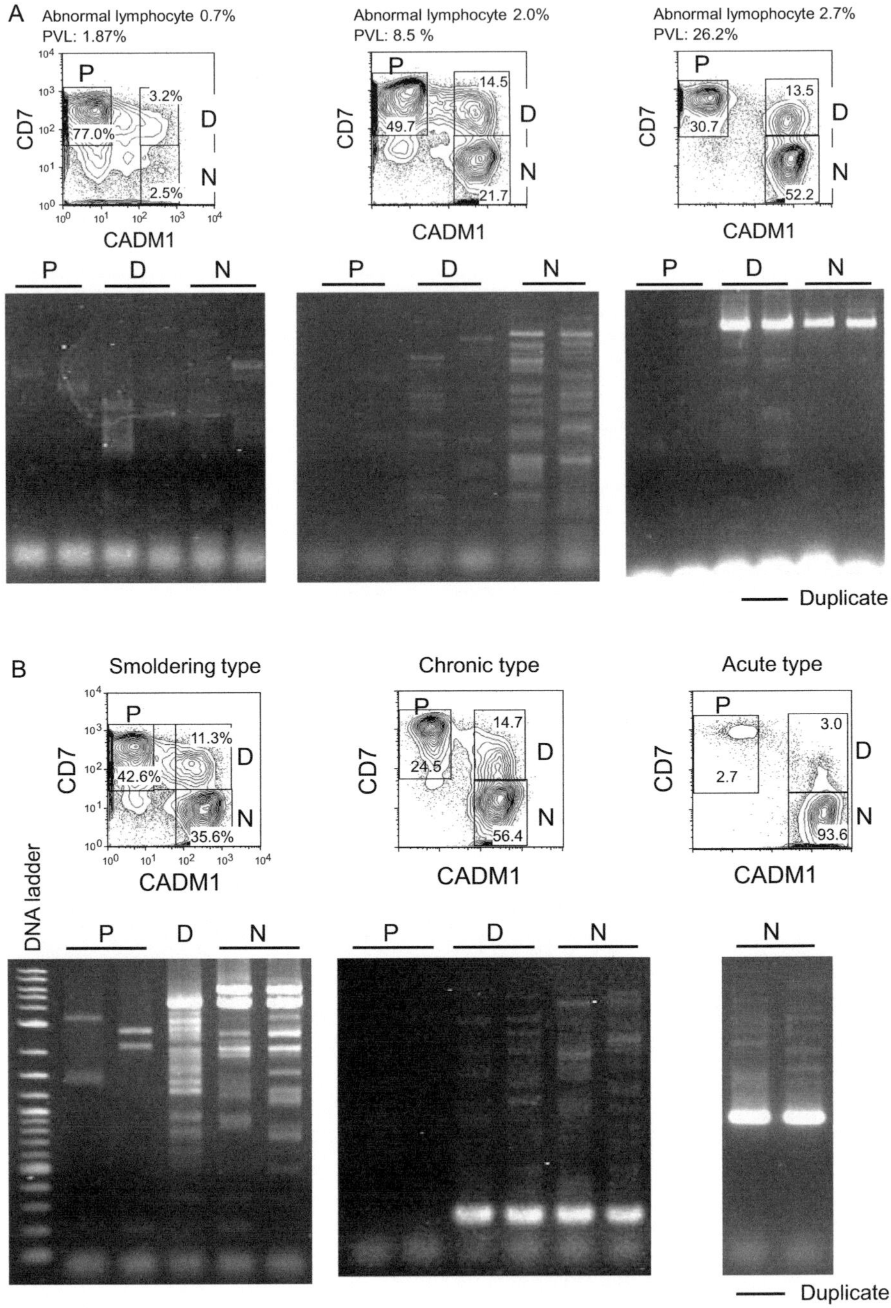


**Fig. 5.5** (**a**) Clonality analysis of asymptomatic carriers. (**b**) Clonality analysis of ATL

mycosis fungoides patients lose CD26 expression [77], whereas upregulation of CD26 has been reported in T-cell acute lymphoblastic leukemia and B-cell chronic lymphocytic leukemia [78]. These data suggest that CD26 may be a useful marker for detecting malignant cells, particularly in lymphoid malignancy, although it may also be useful for other malignancies such as melanoma [79] and mesothelioma [80]. Kamihira et al. examined CD26 expression in ATL patients and HTLV-1 asymptomatic carriers and found that CD26 expression was suppressed or lost in ATL cells [81]. The expression level declined along with progression of disease status by promoter methylation of the gene. The same group further investigated the proportion of CD26-positive cells along with those of CD7, CD25, and CCR4 in the peripheral blood from asymptomatic carriers to indolent ATL (smoldering- and chronic-type) patients [82]. The downregulation of CD26 expression preceded the decrease in CD7 expression and upregulation of CD25 and CCR4 expression as asymptomatic carriers progressed into indolent ATL. They revealed that the CD26/CD25 ratio was a specific and sensitive surrogate marker for the detection of the clonal status of cells infected with HTLV-1. This is important considering that there are asymptomatic carriers who exhibit an oligoclonal pattern of cells infected with HTLV-1, and similarly, smoldering ATL is heterogeneous in the clonality of cells infected with HTLV-1 [70].

## 5.8 Conclusions

ATL is a malignancy of CD4(+) T cells, but some cases express CD8 and may lose CD4 expression. Among pan-T markers, ATL cells express CD2, CD3, and CD5, but usually lack CD7. They express CD25, which is the $\alpha$ chain of the IL-2 receptor and an activated T cell marker. Regarding chemokine receptors, they express CCR1, CCR4, CCR7, CCR8, CCR10, and CXCR4. This immunophenotypic profile resembles those of Th2 cells and Treg cells. In fact, ATL cells express Treg markers, such as GITR and CTLA4. Furthermore, ATL cells express FoxP3, the master regulator of Treg cells. These data suggest that ATL cells may originate from Tregs, but FoxP3 is induced by HBZ and the Treg phenotype can be induced by FoxP3. The origin of ATL cells should be determined in the future. ATL cells paradoxically express CADM1, a tumor suppressor gene of many cancers. Cells infected with HTLV-1 acquire CADM1 expression along with oncogenesis into ATL. Furthermore, cells infected with HTLV-1 gradually lose expression of CD7 and CD26 in the oncogenic process and downregulate CD3 expression. These immunophenotypical changes are useful for analyzing oncogenesis in cells infected with HTLV-1. The typical immunophenotype of ATL cells is summarized in Table 5.1.

**Table 5.1** Typical immunophenotype of ATL cells

| *Typically/frequently positive markers on ATL cells* | |
|---|---|
| Pan-T cell markers | CD2, CD3, CD5 |
| Activation markers | CD25 |
| Chemokine receptors | CCR1, CCR4, CCR7, CCR8, CCR10, CXCR4 |
| Regulatory T cell-related markers | CTLA4, GITR |
| Death receptors | CD95 (Fas), TRAIL receptor |
| Others | CD45RO, CD71 (transferrin receptor), CADM1 |

| *Usually negative markers on ATL cells* | |
|---|---|
| Pan-T cell markers | CD7 |
| Chemokine receptors | CCR2, CCR3, CCR5, CCR8, CCR6, CCR9, CXCR1, CXCR2 |
| | CXCR3, CXCR5 |
| Others | CD45RA, CD26 |

# References


1. Ohshima, K., Jafe, E.S. and Kikuchi M. Adult T-cell leukemia/lymphoma. In: WHO classification of tumors of haematopoietic and lymphoid tissues. Lyon: IARC; 2008. p. 281–4.
2. Went P, et al. Marker expression in peripheral T-cell lymphoma: a proposed clinical-pathologic prognostic score. J Clin Oncol. 2006;24(16):2472–9.
3. Klemke CD, et al. Histopathological and immunophenotypical criteria for the diagnosis of Sézary syndrome in differentiation from other erythrodermic skin diseases: a European Organisation for Research and Treatment of Cancer (EORTC) Cutaneous Lymphoma Task Force Study of 97 cases. Br J Dermatol. 2015;173(1):93–105.
4. Kamihira S, et al. Phenotypical diversity and prognosis of adult T-cell leukemia. Leuk Res. 1992;16(5):435–41.
5. Ramirez F, et al. Glucocorticoids induce the expression of CD8c chains on concanavalin A-activated rat CD4 + T cells: induction is inhibited by rat recombinant interleukin 4. J Exp Med. 1992;176(6):1551–9.
6. Yamada Y, et al. Established IL-2-dependent double-negative (CD4- CD8-) TCR alpha beta/CD3+ ATL cells: induction of CD4 expression. Br J Haematol. 1994;88(2):234–41.
7. Yaamada Y. Phenotypic and functional analysis of leukemic cells from 16 patients with adult T-cell leukemia/lymphoma. Blood. 1993;61(1):192–9.
8. Fazekas de St Groth B, Smith AL, Higgins CA. T cell activation: in vivo veritas. Immunol Cell Biol. 2004;82(3):260–8.
9. Shimabukuro-Vornhagen A, et al. Activated human B cells: stimulatory or tolerogenic antigen-presenting cells? Blood. 2009;114:746–7.
10. Triplett TA, et al. Defining a functionally distinct subset of human memory CD4+ T cells that are CD25POS and FOXP3NEG. Eur J Immunol. 2012;42(7):1893–905.
11. Sakaguchi S. Regulatory T cells: history and perspective. Methods Mol Biol. 2011;707:3–17.
12. Yodoi J, Maeda M. Discovery of ATL: an odyssey in restrospect. Int J Hematol. 2011;94(5):423–8.
13. Turturro F. Denileukin diftitox: a biotherapeutic paradigm shift in the treatment of lymphoid-derived disorders. Expert Rev Anticancer Ther. 2007;7(1):11–7.
14. Tobinai K. Clinical trials for human T-cell lymphotropic virus type I-associated peripheral T-cell lymphoma in Japan. Semin Hematol. 2010;47(Suppl 1):S5–7.

15. Berkowitz JL, et al. Safety, efficacy, and pharmacokinetics/pharmacodynamics of daclizumab (anti-CD25) in patients with adult T-cell leukemia/lymphoma. Clin Immunol. 2014;155(2): 176–87.
16. Kreitman RJ, et al. Phase I trial of recombinant immunotoxin anti-Tac(Fv)-PE38 (LMB-2) in patients with hematologic malignancies. J Clin Oncol. 2000;18(8):1622–36.
17. Kreitman RJ, et al. Complete remissions of adult T-cell leukemia with anti-CD25 recombinant immunotoxin LMB-2 and chemotherapy to block immunogenicity. Clin Cancer Res. 2015;22: 310–8.
18. Hanafusa T, et al. Flow cytometric immunophenotyping of adult T-cell leukemia/lymphoma using CD3 gating. Am J Clin Pathol. 2005;124(2):199–204.
19. Akl H, et al. HTLV-I infection of WE17/10 CD4+ cell line leads to progressive alteration of Ca2+ influx that eventually results in loss of CD7 expression and activation of an antiapoptotic pathway involving AKT and BAD which paves the way for malignant transformation. Leukemia. 2007;21(4):788–96.
20. Akl H, et al. Progressive loss of CD3 expression after HTLV-I infection results from chromatin remodeling affecting all the CD3 genes and persists despite early viral genes silencing. Virol J. 2007;4:85.
21. Tian Y, et al. Leukemic T cells are specifically enriched in a unique CD3(dim) CD7(low) subpopulation of CD4(+) T cells in acute-type adult T-cell leukemia. Cancer Sci. 2011; 102(3):569–77.
22. Zlotnik A, Yoshie O, Nomiyama H. The chemokine and chemokine receptor superfamilies and their molecular evolution. Genome Biol. 2006;7(12):243.
23. Griffith JW, Sokol CL, Luster AD. Chemokines and chemokine receptors: positioning cells for host defense and immunity. Annu Rev Immunol. 2014;32:659–702.
24. Imai T, et al. Selective recruitment of CCR4-bearing Th2 cells toward antigen-presenting cells by the CC chemokines thymus and activation-regulated chemokine and macrophage-derived chemokine. Int J Immunol. 1999;11(1):81–8.
25. Curiel TJ, et al. Specific recruitment of regulatory T cells in ovarian carcinoma fosters immune privilege and predicts reduced survival. Nat Med. 2004;10(9):942–9.
26. Takashi Ishida AU, Iida S, et al. Clinical significance of CCR4 expression in adult T-cell leukemia/lymphoma: its close association with skin involvement and unfavorable outcome. Clin Cancer Res. 2003;9(10):3625–34.
27. Ohshima K, et al. Classification of distinct subtypes of peripheral T-cell lymphoma unspecified, identified by chemokine and chemokine receptor expression: analysis of prognosis. Int J Oncol. 2004;25(3):605–13.
28. Ishii T, et al. Defucosylated humanized anti-CCR4 monoclonal antibody KW-0761 as a novel immunotherapeutic agent for adult T-cell leukemia/lymphoma. Clin Cancer Res. 2010;16(5): 1520–31.
29. Ishida T, et al. Defucosylated anti-CCR4 monoclonal antibody (KW-0761) for relapsed adult T-cell leukemia-lymphoma: a multicenter phase II study. J Clin Oncol. 2012;30(8):837–42.
30. Ishida T, et al. Dose-intensified chemotherapy alone or in combination with mogamulizumab in newly diagnosed aggressive adult T-cell leukaemia-lymphoma: a randomized phase II study. Br J Haematol. 2015;169(5):672–82.
31. Ruckes T, et al. Autocrine antiapoptotic stimulation of cultured adultT-cell leukemia cells by overexpression of the chemokine I-309. Blood. 2001;98(4):1150–9.
32. Hasegawa H, et al. Increased chemokine receptor CCR7/EBI1 expression enhances the infiltration of lymphoid organs by adult T-cell leukemia cells. Blood. 2000;95(1):30–8.
33. Harasawa H, et al. Survey of chemokine receptor expression reveals frequent co-expression of skin-homing CCR4 and CCR10 in adult T-cell leukemia/lymphoma. Leuk Lymphoma. 2006;47(10):2163–73.
34. Horikawa T, et al. IFN-gamma-inducible expression of thymus and activation-regulated chemokine/CCL17 and macrophage-derived chemokine/CCL22 in epidermal keratinocytes and their roles in atopic dermatitis. Int Immunol. 2002;14(7):767–73.

35. Wang W, et al. Identification of a novel chemokine (CCL28), which binds CCR10 (GPR2). J Biol Chem. 2000;275(29):22313–23.
36. Pan J, et al. Cutting edge: a novel chemokine ligand for CCR10 and CCR3 expressed by epithelial cells in mucosal tissues. J Immunol. 2000;165(6):2943–9.
37. Sakaguchi S, et al. FOXP3+ regulatory T cells in the human immune system. Nat Rev Immunol. 2010;10(7):490–500.
38. Ronchetti S, et al. Glucocorticoid-induced tumour necrosis factor receptor-related protein: a key marker of functional regulatory T cells. J Immunol Res. 2015;2015:171520.
39. Takahashi T, et al. Immunologic self-tolerance maintained by CD25(+)CD4(+) regulatory T cells constitutively expressing cytotoxic T lymphocyte–associated antigen 4. J Exp Med. 2000;192(2):303–9.
40. Kohno T, et al. Possible origin of adult T-cell leukemia/lymphoma cells from human T lymphotropic virus type-1-infected regulatory T cells. Cancer Sci. 2005;96(8):527–33.
41. Matsubara Y, et al. Phenotypic and functional relationship between adult T-cell leukemia cells and regulatory T cells. Leukemia. 2005;19(3):482–3.
42. Ohkura N, Kitagawa Y, Sakaguchi S. Development and maintenance of regulatory T cells. Immunity. 2013;38(3):414–23.
43. Karube K, et al. Expression of FoxP3, a key molecule in CD4CD25 regulatory T cells, in adult T-cell leukaemia/lymphoma cells. Br J Haematol. 2004;126(1):81–4.
44. Satou Y, et al. HTLV-1 modulates the frequency and phenotype of FoxP3 + CD4+ T cells in virus-infected individuals. Retrovirology. 2012;9:46.
45. Gaudray G, et al. The complementary strand of the human T-cell leukemia virus type 1 RNA genome encodes a bZIP transcription factor that down-regulates viral transcription. J Virol. 2002;76(24):12813–22.
46. Satou Y, et al. HTLV-1 bZIP factor induces T-cell lymphoma and systemic inflammation in vivo. PLoS Pathog. 2011;7(2):e1001274.
47. Schneider YJ, et al. The role of receptor-mediated endocytosis in iron metabolism. Prog Clin Biol Res. 1982;91:495–521.
48. Trowbridge IS, Shackelford DA. Structure and function of transferrin receptors and their relationship to cell growth. Biochem Soc Symp. 1986;51:117–29.
49. Gatter KC, et al. Transferrin receptors in human tissues: their distribution and possible clinical relevance. J Clin Pathol. 1983;36(5):539–45.
50. Vidal C, et al. Human T lymphotropic virus I infection deregulates surface expression of the transferrin receptor. J Immunol. 1988;141(3):984–8.
51. Moura IC, et al. Aneutralizing monoclonal antibody (mAbA24) directed against the transferrin receptor induces apoptosis of tumor T lymphocytes from ATL patients. Blood. 2004;103 (5):1838–45.
52. Yamazaki J, et al. Identification of cancer stem cells in a Tax-transgenic (Tax-Tg) mouse model of adult T-cell leukemia/lymphoma. Blood. 2009;114(13):2709–20.
53. Yonehara S, et al. A cell-killing monoclonal antibody (ANTI-Fas) to a cell surface antigen co-downregulated with the receptor of tumor necrosis factor. J Exp Med. 1989;169(5):1747–56.
54. Kamihira S, et al. Quantitative characterization and potential function of membrane Fas/APO-1 (CD95) receptors on leukaemic cells from chronic B and T lymphoid leukaemias. Br J Haematol. 1997;99(4):858–65.
55. Krueger A, et al. HTLV-1Tax protects against CD95-mediated apoptosis by induction of the cellular FLICE-inhibitory protein (c-FLIP). Blood. 2006;107(10):3933–9.
56. Okamoto K, et al. Human T-cell leukemia virus type-I oncoprotein Tax inhibits Fas-mediated apoptosis by inducing cellular FLIP through activation of NF-kappaB. Genes Cells. 2006;11(2):177–91.
57. Wang W, et al. Human T-cell leukemia virus type 1 Tax-deregulated autophagy pathway and c-FLIP expression contribute to resistance against death receptor-mediated apoptosis. J Virol. 2014;88(5):2786–98.

58. Maeda T, et al. Fas gene mutation in the progression of adult T cell leukemia. J Exp Med. 1999;189(7):1063–71.
59. Sugahara K, et al. Soluble and membrane isoforms of Fas/CD95 in fresh adult T-cell leukemia (ATL) cells and ATL-cell lines. Int J Cancer. 1997;72(1):128–32.
60. Safa AR. c-FLIP, a master anti-apoptotic regulator. Exp Oncol. 2012;34(3):176–84.
61. Ashkenazi A, Dixit VM. Apoptosis control by death and decoy receptors. Curr Opin Cell Biol. 1999;11(2):255–60.
62. Hasegawa H, et al. Sensitivity of adult T-cell leukaemia lymphoma cells to tumour necrosis factor-related apoptosis-inducing ligand. Br J Haematol. 2005;128(2):253–65.
63. Ding J, et al. Wogonin and related natural flavones overcome tumor necrosis factor-related apoptosis-inducing ligand (TRAIL) protein resistance of tumors by down-regulation of c-FLIP protein and up-regulation of TRAIL receptor 2 expression. J Biol Chem. 2012;287(1):641–9.
64. Murakami Y. Involvement of a cell adhesion molecule, TSLC1/IGSF4, in human oncogenesis. Cancer Sci. 2005;96(9):543–52.
65. Galibert L, et al. Nectin-like protein 2 defines a subset of T-cell zone dendritic cells and is a ligand for class-I-restricted T-cell-associated molecule. J Biol Chem. 2005;280(23):21955–64.
66. Watabe K, et al. IGSF4: a new intercellular adhesion molecule that is called by three names, TSLC1, SgIGSF and SynCAM, by virtue of its diverse function. Histol Histopathol. 2003;18(4):1321–9.
67. Sasaki H, et al. Overexpression of a cell adhesion molecule, TSLC1, as a possible molecular marker for acute-type adult T-cell leukemia. Blood. 2005;105(3):1204–13.
68. Nakahata S, et al. Clinical significance of CADM1/TSLC1/IgSF4 expression in adult T-cell leukemia/lymphoma. Leukemia. 2012;26(6):1238–46.
69. Nakahata S, et al. CADM1/TSLC1 is a novel cell surface marker for adult T-cell leukemia/ lymphoma. J Clin Exp Hematop. 2012;52(1):17–22.
70. Kobayashi S, et al. CADM1 expression and stepwise downregulation of CD7 are closely associated with clonal expansion of HTLV-I-infected cells in adult T-cell leukemia/lymphoma. Clin Cancer Res. 2014;20(11):2851–61.
71. Yamagishi M, et al. Polycomb-mediated loss of miR-31 activates NIK-dependent NF-kappaB pathway in adult T cell leukemia and other cancers. Cancer Cell. 2012;21(1):121–35.
72. Asanuma S, et al. Adult T-cell leukemia cells are characterized by abnormalities of Helios expression that promote T cell growth. Cancer Sci. 2013;104(8):1097–106.
73. Takahashi R, et al. Epigenetic deregulation of Ellis Van Creveld confers robust Hedgehog signaling in adult T-cell leukemia. Cancer Sci. 2014;105(9):1160–9.
74. Kobayashi S, et al. Advanced human T-cell leukemia virus type 1 carriers and early-stage indolent adult T-cell leukemia-lymphoma are indistinguishable based on CADM1 positivity in flow cytometry. Cancer Sci. 2015;106(5):598–603.
75. Iwata S, et al. CD26/dipeptidyl peptidase IV in context: the different roles of a multifunctional ectoenzyme in malignant transformation. J Exp Med. 1999;190(3):301–5.
76. Ohnuma K, Dang NH, Morimoto C. Revisiting an old acquaintance: CD26 and its molecular mechanisms in T cell function. Trends Immunol. 2008;29(6):295–301.
77. Jones D, et al. Absence of CD26 expression is a useful marker for diagnosis of T-cell lymphoma in peripheral' blood. Am J Clin Pathol. 2001;115(6):885–92.
78. Bauvois B, et al. Constitutive expression of CD26/dipeptidylpeptidase IV on peripheral blood B lymphocytes of patients with B chronic lymphocytic leukaemia. Br J Cancer. 1999;79(7/8):1042–8.
79. Morrison ME, et al. A marker for neoplastic progression of human melanocytes is a cell surface ectopeptidase. J Exp Med. 1993;177(4):1135–43.
80. Amatya VJ, et al. Overexpression of CD26/DPPIV in mesothelioma tissue and mesothelioma cell lines. Oncol Rep. 2011;26(6):1369–75.
81. Tsuji T, et al. Clinical and oncologic implications in epigenetic down-regulation of CD26/ dipeptidyl peptidase IV in adult T-cell leukemia cells. Int J Hematol. 2004;80(3):254–60.
82. Kamihira S, et al. Heterogeneity in clonal nature in the smoldering subtype of adult T-cell leukemia: continuity from carrier status to smoldering ATL. Int J Hematol. 2012;95(4): 399–408.

# Chapter 6
# Leukemogenesis and Molecular Characteristics of Tumor Cells

Toshiki Watanabe

## 6.1 Introduction

Adult T-cell leukemia (ATL) is caused by human T-cell leukemia virus (HTLV-1) [1, 2]. ATL develops after a long clinical latency of about 50 or more years after mother-to-child infection and is classified into four clinical subtypes: smoldering, chronic, acute, and lymphoma [3]. ATL cells are monoclonally expanded HTLV-1-infected cells with malignant transformation. However, whether ATL develops after horizontal transmission by sexual contact or blood transfusion remains unclear. Conversely, as described in detail in the following sections, asymptomatic HTLV-1 carriers have also been shown to have clonally expanded HTLV-1-infected cells in peripheral blood. Thus, the malignant transformation of a limited number of cells among the immortalized and clonally expanded HTLV-1-infected cells is suggested to result in the apparent monoclonal growth and onset of ATL. This process is based on the accumulation of five or more genetic events, thus fitting with the multistep carcinogenesis model [4]. HTLV-1 infection, followed by the expression of viral gene products in infected cells, is considered to be among the early events that determine the fate of infected T cells.

In this chapter, we summarize the cellular and molecular characteristics of ATL cells. We particularly focus on the clonal growth, cellular and molecular characteristics, and genomic and epigenomic abnormalities with aberrant gene expression profiles of HTLV-1-infected cells and ATL cells. Full understanding of the processes underlying immortalization, clonal proliferation, and malignant transformation is not yet complete. Questions that remain to be answered include the following:

T. Watanabe (✉)
Department of Medical Genome Sciences, Graduate School of Frontier Sciences, The University of Tokyo, Tokyo, Japan
e-mail: tnabe@marianna-u.ac.jp



T. Watanabe, T. Fukushima (eds.), *Adult T-cell Leukemia/Lymphoma*,
DOI 10.1007/978-4-431-56523-9_6

1. How and when are virus-infected cells immortalized?
2. How is the size of HTLV-1-infected clones regulated?
3. What are the genetic and/or epigenetic mechanisms that determine the differences between immortalization and transformation?
4. Which genes are involved in the phenotypic progression of HTLV-1-infected T cells?

The information summarized in this chapter will aid in the understanding of the molecular mechanisms underlying the leukemogenesis of ATL and provide clues for designing molecularly targeted therapies against ATL.

## 6.2 Clonal Growth of HTLV-1-Infected T Cells

### *6.2.1 Clonality of ATL Cells*

Soon after the discovery of HTLV-1, clonal growth of ATL cells was demonstrated by Southern blot analysis using HTLV-1 provirus DNA as a probe [5, 6]. The results clearly showed that ATL cells were monoclonally expanded HTLV-1-infected cells. A part of the patients were shown to have a monoclonal tumor cells harboring two or more integrated proviruses by analysis of T-cell receptor β-chain rearrangement and the observation of multiple bands by Southern blotting.

The next set of studies determined whether ATL patients could simultaneously have multiple clones of HTLV-1-infected cells. Some case reports provided suggestive evidence for the presence of multiple clones in vivo at certain time points or during the clinical course. Examples include a chronic ATL patient with concomitant $CD4^{+}/CD8^{-}$ and $CD4^{-}CD8^{+}$ clones [7], a patient with two independent clones in the peripheral blood and lymph nodes [8], a patient with the emergence of a new clone after spontaneous remission [9], and a patient with a giant skin tumor harboring five independent clones [10]. Clonal exchange during the clinical course was also reported in another study [11]. Taken together, these data suggested that multiple clones could be concurrently undergoing transformation in an individual and that two or more fully transformed clones could occasionally coexist.

Using array comparative genomic hybridization (CGH), Seto and colleagues analyzed paired samples from the peripheral blood and lymph nodes of patients with acute-type ATL. They demonstrated that these patients contained multiple subclones with distinct genomic aberrations. In many ATL cases, multiple subclones in the lymph nodes have been found to originate from a common clone, often with a specific lymph node subclone found in the peripheral blood [12, 13]. Collectively, these reports strongly suggest the presence of clones concurrently undergoing transformation in vivo (Fig. 6.1).

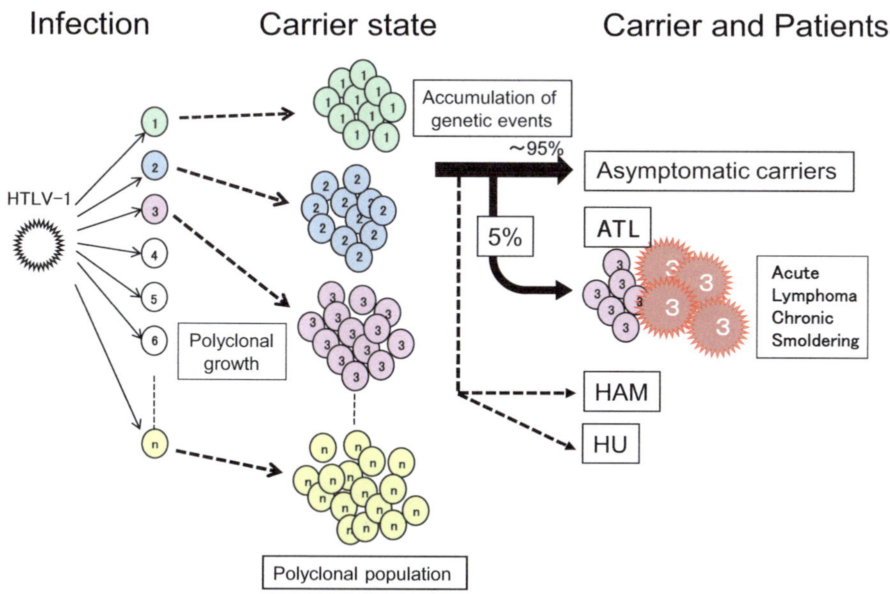


**Fig. 6.1** Clonality of human T-cell leukemia virus 1-infected T cells in different clinical stages. A schematic presentation of clonal growth of human T-cell leukemia virus 1 (HTLV-1)-infected T cells shows the polyclonal nature of HTLV-1-infected cells in carriers, consisting of varying numbers of immortalized cells. Each clone originates from a single infected T cell. Accumulation of genetic events leads to the progression and transformation of a subset of cells resulting in the onset of adult T-cell leukemia (ATL). ATL cells are members of specific clones that have been malignantly transformed. *HTLV-1* human T-cell leukemia virus 1, *ATL* adult T-cell leukemia/lymphoma, *HAM* HTLV-1-associated myelopathy, *HU* HTLV-1 uveitis

### *6.2.2 Clonality of HTLV-1-Infected T Cells in Carriers*

Given that ATL cells result from the clonal expansion of HTLV-1-infected T cells that undergo malignant transformation, the next question pertains to the clonality of infected T cells in asymptomatic carriers in vivo. Matsuoka and colleagues utilized inverse polymerase chain reaction (iPCR) to address this question [14]. They demonstrated that iPCR could quickly detect clonally integrated HTLV-1 proviral DNA in samples from ATL patients. They also showed that iPCR could detect multiple amplified bands consisting of HTLV-1 proviral and flanking cellular DNA, demonstrating the polyclonal nature of HTLV-1-infected cells in asymptomatic carriers. This technique has been widely applied to characterize the clonality of HTLV-1 infected cells in various clinical settings [15–17]. Okayama et al. reported a difference in the stability of clonality depending on the mode of virus transmission. The clonality of adult seroconverters who appeared to have acquired the virus horizontally from their spouses was more heterogeneous and less stable than that of long-term carriers who had most likely been infected through breastfeeding in their infancy [18, 19].

Wattel et al. employed linker-mediated PCR (LMPCR) to analyze integration sites of the HTLV-1 provirus. LMPCR was more sensitive, allowing detection of a greater number of integrated proviruses [20, 21]. Carriers with strongyloidiasis showed oligoclonal expansion of HTLV-1-infected cells and high proviral loads [22]. These new techniques provided information on the clonality of HTLV-1-infected cells in various clinical conditions.

Subsequently, Bangham and colleagues developed a novel, high-throughput protocol using next-generation sequencing (NGS) to map and quantify proviral genomic integration sites. They revealed that there were between 10,000 and 100,000 clones in the peripheral blood of HTLV-1-infected individuals, which was much higher than previously speculated [23]. They also claimed that HTLV-1 integration into the host genome was not random and that it was associated with specific transcription factor binding sites [24]. They also suggested that integration of HTLV-1 upstream of certain proto-oncogenes was associated with ATL [25]. Although information revealed by this new approach significantly impacted the understanding on the clonality of infected T cells in vivo, this technique was limited in determining the number of infected cells. This approach depended on the size variation of sheared genomic DNA fragments that were a maximum of 400 base pairs as the size of recovered DNA fragments was distributed between 300 and 700 base pairs following shearing. To overcome this limitation, Firouzi et al. introduced oligomer tags of eight nucleotides that marked sheared DNA before amplification, which enabled the discrimination of more than 60,000 cells, dramatically expanding the ability to quantify cells with this technique [26].

The results of these analyses provided firm evidence supporting the hypothesis that HTLV-1 carriers harbor a great number of HTLV-1-infected and immortalized clones and that each clone originates from a single infected T cell. The size of cell populations belonging to specific clones (clone sizes) also varied greatly, and some clones had large populations that could be detected as clonal expansion by conventional techniques, such as Southern blot hybridization and iPCR.

One other issue related to HTLV-1-infected T cells in vivo is the identification of HTLV-1-infected cells among uninfected T cells. Uchimaru and colleagues developed a technique using multicolor fluorescence-activated cell sorting (FACS) to identify infected cells and discriminate between untransformed and transformed HTLV-1-infected CD4$^+$ lymphocytes based on the cell surface expression of CD7 and CADM-1 (TSLC1) [27, 28]. A combination of the abovementioned techniques will provide detailed information on the number and cellular characteristics of HTLV-1-infected cells in carriers and in patients with HTLV-1-associated diseases.

## 6.3 Molecular Characteristics of ATL Cells

### 6.3.1 *mRNA Expression*

ATL cells have been extensively documented to express cytokines, chemokines, their receptors, and adhesion molecules, most of which have also been shown to be targeted by the viral transactivator protein Tax [29–33]. Morishita and colleagues reported that

CADM1, a cell surface molecule originally isolated as a tumor suppressor in non-small cell lung cancer [34], was highly expressed in ATL cells [35]. Subsequently, CADM1 was shown to be expressed not only in transformed ATL cells but also in HTLV-1-infected non-transformed T cells in carriers. CADM1 is currently used for the identification of HTLV-1-infected T cells by multicolor FACS analysis as described above [27, 28]. Other highly expressed molecules include PTHrP and other markers that are not expressed in normal T cells but play important roles in the unique pathophysiology of ATL. PTHrP is responsible for humoral hypercalcemia of malignancy (HHM) that occasionally accompanies solid cancers. In ATL, HHM is observed during the clinical course of more than half of the patients and was one of the major causes of mortality until therapy for HHM was established [36].

The overexpression of cell adhesion molecules and chemokine receptors [30–33, 37–40] and aberrant expression of these genes may be a source of organ infiltration of ATL cells. One intriguing aspect of these data is the expression of genes that are not normally expressed in T cells [41, 42]. Lineage-independent ectopic expression of many genes characterizes ATL cells and suggests underlying abnormalities in epigenetic regulation that determines tissue-specific gene expression.

### 6.3.2 MicroRNA Expression

To date, only four studies have characterized microRNA (miRNA) expression profiles in HTLV-1/ATL cell lines and ATL patients. Pichler et al. reported that *miR-21*, *miR-24*, *miR-146a*, and *miR-155* were upregulated, whereas *miR-223* was downregulated in HTLV-1-transformed cells. They showed that *miR-146a* expression was induced by HTLV-1 Tax and NF-κB signaling [43]. Bellon et al. analyzed ATL cells and control samples from HTLV-1 negative donors using microarray and demonstrated the downregulation of *miR-181a*, *miR-132*, and *miR-125a* and upregulation of *miR-155* and *miR-142-3p*. They also reported that *miR-150* and *miR-223* were differentially expressed in vitro and in vivo. Both *miR-150* and *miR-223* were upregulated in uncultured ATL cells and downregulated in HTLV-1-transformed cell lines [44].

Yeung et al. studied miRNA expression profiles in ATL cells obtained from acute-type ATL patients and in ATL-derived cell lines. Among miRNAs that were differentially expressed, six miRNAs were upregulated in ATL cells, and of these, *miR-93* and *miR-130b* were shown to target TP53INP1. The low levels of TP53INP1 detected in ATL cells were upregulated by the addition of an antagomir [45]. Yamagishi et al. investigated the miRNA expression signature in primary ATL cells using 40 ATL samples and $CD4^+$ T cells from 22 age-adjusted healthy volunteers. They found that the vast majority of differentially expressed miRNAs were downregulated in primary ATL cells. Furthermore, among significantly downregulated miRNAs, the most severely suppressed was *miR-31*, which was nearly undetectable. They also identified *NIK* as a target of *miR-31* and showed that the deficiency of *miR-31* resulted in overexpression of *NIK* that led to the constitutive activation of the NF-κB pathway [46].

### 6.3.3 *Signal Transduction*

Expression of HTLV-1 Tax induces various signaling pathways, many of which are also observed in primary ATL cells. The best known example is the NF-κB pathway, which is constitutively active in ATL cells. This pathway has been shown to underlie uncontrolled growth and apoptosis resistance [47]. Inhibition of NF-κB by a selective inhibitor, dehydroxymethylepoxyquinomicin (DHMEQ), has been documented to induce apoptosis of ATL cells and specifically reduce the number of HTLV-1-infected T cells in asymptomatic carriers [48]. One of the demonstrated mechanisms underlying NF-κB activation is the suppression of *miR-31* overexpression, leading to NIK and NF-κB activation [46]. In addition, the activation-inducible lymphocyte immunomediatory molecule (AILIM)/inducible costimulator (ICOS) signaling has been shown to be responsible for the constitutive activation of phosphoinositide-3 (PI3)-kinase/AKT cascade in ATL cells, inducing the formation of multi-lobulated nuclei observed in ATL [49]. Furthermore, the Jak/STAT pathway has been shown to become activated in ATL cells and in this case was associated with leukemic cell proliferation [50].

There is limited information on other signal transduction pathways that may be involved in primary ATL cells, although HTLV-1 Tax has been shown to activate the MAPK pathway in vitro.

## 6.4 Genomic Abnormalities

### 6.4.1 *Cytogenetic Characteristics*

ATL cells exhibit a variety of cytogenetic abnormalities; however, specific recombination or amplification/deletion events have not been cytogenetically identified. Kamada et al. reported the results of a cytogenetic study including 107 ATL patients and found that clonal chromosome abnormalities were found in 96% of the cases. A variety of numerical and structural abnormalities were also found; however, none of these were ATL specific [51].

Itoyama et al. studied the relation between chromosomal abnormalities and clinical outcomes in 50 ATL cases. They found certain chromosomal aberrations to be correlated with one or more of the clinical features as well as the clinical severity. Multiple breaks (at least six) correlated with shorter survival [52]. CGH analysis of 64 cases also revealed a correlation with the clinical course. The most frequent aberrations included gains at chromosomes 14q, 7q, and 3p and losses at chromosomes 6q and 13q. Chromosomal imbalances, losses, and gains were more frequently observed in aggressive ATL cases than in indolent ATL cases. Analyses of sequential samples during progression suggested clonal changes at crisis; clonal diversity was common during progression to ATL, and CGH alterations were associated with the clinical course [53].

### 6.4.2 Specific Genetic Abnormalities

Tumor suppressor genes are essential for controlling cellular proliferation, inducing apoptosis, linking DNA damage signals to cell cycle arrest checkpoints, and activating appropriate DNA repair pathways. Thus, the inactivation of tumor suppressors by somatic mutations or epigenetic mechanisms is frequently reported in many cancer types and is suggested to be involved in tumor initiation and development.

There are many reports on the inactivation of tumor suppressor genes involved in cell cycle checkpoints that may lead to the uncontrolled proliferation of ATL cells. Mutations in *TP53* have been reported in about 30% of ATL cases [54–57] in contrast to its observation in less than 3% of non-HTLV-1-associated T-cell neoplasms [58]. Functional inactivation of p53 has also been reported in ATL cells [59–61]. Although the viral oncoprotein Tax has been shown to inactivate the transcriptional functions of p53 [62–66], the underlying mechanisms of p53 inactivation are not known as viral protein Tax is not expressed in ATL cells [67].

In many human cancers, *CDKN2A* (*p14ARF* and *p16INK4a*) is frequently mutated, deleted, or inactivated through promoter hypermethylation [68, 69]. Homozygous deletion or promoter hypermethylation of *CDKN2A* has been observed in at least 20% of acute ATL patients, whereas the loss of *CDKN2A* is infrequent in chronic and smoldering ATL cases [70–72].

The expression of *CDKN1A* (*p21CIP1/WAF1*) is frequently downregulated in acute ATL cases due to hypermethylation of the promoter region. Watanabe et al. reported that promoter methylation was observed in 95% of the ATL patients analyzed, with hypermethylation and partial methylation found in about 25% and 70% of the cases, respectively [73].

A study suggested that *RB1* is infrequently mutated or deleted in ATL tumor cells [55]. Another study reported on the homozygous loss of exon 1 in 5% of ATL patients, whereas no point mutations were found [74]. In addition, mutations of *RB2/p130* were found in approximately 2.5% of ATL patients [75, 76]. In another study, ATL cells were documented as expressing low levels of *RB1* in about 50% of ATL patients, and the posttranscriptional regulation of *RB1* was hypothesized [76]. Additionally, low levels of Rb expression have been reported to correlate with poor prognosis and shorter survival [77].

SHP1 is implicated in the degradation of PIP3 and inhibition of the PI3K/AKT pathway [78]. *SHP1* has been found to be hypermethylated in 90% of the ATL patients. Inactivation by DNA methylation is more frequently observed in aggressive-type ATL [79]. No mutations have been identified in the *H-*, *N-*, *and K-Ras or c-Myc* genes [55].

### 6.4.3 Comprehensive Analysis of Genomic Abnormalities

Comprehensive analyses of gene expression (transcriptome analysis) of ATL cells have been conducted by several groups. Morishita and colleagues found that *CADM1*, which was overexpressed in ATL cells, was involved in interactions with vascular endothelial cells [35]. They demonstrated that CADM1 is a cell surface marker of ATL [80]. CADM1 expression has also been confirmed to be a marker of HTLV-1-infected immortalized T cells and has been used in multicolor FACS analysis to identify these cells in vivo [27]. Asanuma et al. reported the expression of alternatively spliced Helios variants, some of which were specific to ATL cells. One of the variants played a role in the proliferation of ATL cells [81].

Ogawa and colleagues reported the results of an integrated genomic and transcriptomic analysis in a cohort of 426 ATL cases [67]. This study, with a massive amount of genomic, methylomic, and transcriptomic data, coupled with cell-based experiments, provided comprehensive and detailed information to gain insight into the pathogenesis of ATL. The data confirmed the deletion and mutation of the viral genome in ATL cells and the lack of expression of the sense strand, including mRNA encoding Tax, in contrast to the constitutive expression of antisense transcript HBZ. Based on the results of whole-genome sequencing and single nucleotide polymorphism array-based copy number analysis, they confirmed the existence of genomic instability that was previously described in ATL. On average, they identified 60 structural variations per sample. Whole-exome sequencing in 81 cases, combined with targeted resequencing of 370 ATL cases, identified 50 genes that were recurrently and significantly mutated, with 13 genes affected in more than 10% of the cases. The most frequently mutated genes in this group were *PLCG1*, *PRKCB*, *CARD11*, and *STAT3*, which are implicated in T-cell receptor (TCR)–NF-κB signaling. In addition, either *CCR4* or *CCR7* was mutated in 40% of ATL cases; *CCR4* mutations were shown to lead to increased PI3K signaling. These data are compatible with the concept of a memory of Tax in the absence of Tax expression in ATL cells (Fig. 6.2).

Accumulation of additional mutations affecting the TCR and NF-κB pathways, together with inactivation of *TP53*, *CDKN2A*, and other mutations, eventually transforms T cells into fully malignant cells. The study by Ogawa and colleagues also showed that ATL cells delete, mutate, or hypermethylate genes encoding components of the class I major histocompatibility complex (MHC), death receptors, and proteins involved in cellular adhesion or immune checkpoints as a strategy to escape detection by the immune system.

The same group recently reported that structural variations (SVs) commonly disrupt the 3′ region of the programmed cell death 1 (*PD-1*) ligand (*PD-L1*) gene in 27% of ATL cases [82]. These SVs invariably led to marked elevations in aberrant PD-L1 transcripts that were stabilized by the truncation of the 3′-untranslated region. This is a unique genetic mechanism of immune escape triggered by SVs since the only known mechanisms for elevated PD-L1 expression is gene

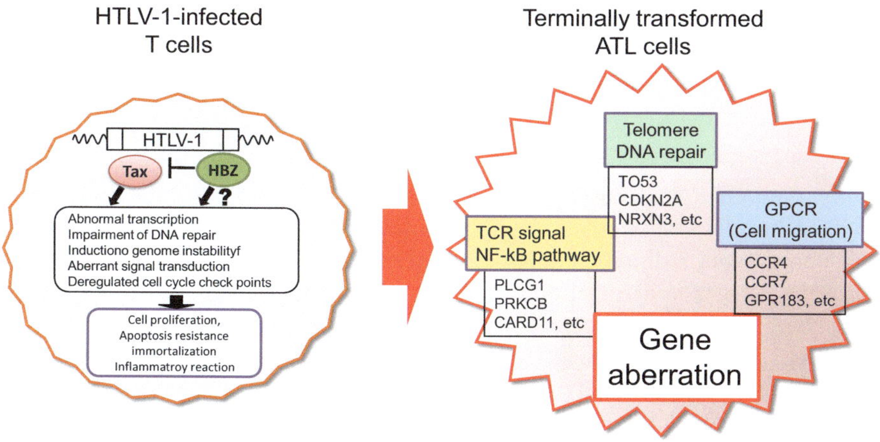


**Fig. 6.2** Accumulation of genomic abnormalities in adult T-cell leukemia cells. In HTLV-1-infected T cells, viral regulatory proteins, Tax and HBZ, are predicted to affect normal cellular functions. After a long latency period, a variety of structural and numerical genomic abnormalities are observed in terminally transformed ATL cells; some of these changes serve the function of Tax, since Tax is not expressed in ATL cells

amplification and utilization of an ectopic promoter by translocation, found in Hodgkin and other B-cell lymphomas and in gastric adenocarcinoma.

Ogawa and colleagues have also reported on the existence of unique *RHOA* mutations in ATL by whole-genome sequencing of an index case, followed by deep sequencing of 203 ATL samples [83]. *RHOA* mutations were found in 15% (30/203) of the samples and were widely distributed across the entire coding sequence but were almost invariably located at the guanosine triphosphate (GTP)-binding pocket. Depending on mutation types and positions, these *RHOA* mutants showed different or even opposite functional consequences related to GTP/guanosine diphosphate (GDP)-binding kinetics, regulation of actin fibers, and transcriptional activation. These findings suggest that both the loss- and gain-of-RHOA functions could be involved in ATL leukemogenesis.

Based on the results of whole-genome NGS using freshly isolated ATL cells, Nicot and colleagues reported the presence of mutations in *SUZ12*, *DNMT1*, *DNMT3A*, *DNMT3B*, *TET1*, *TET2*, *IDH1*, *IDH2*, *MLL*, *MLL2*, *MLL3*, and *MLL4* [84]. *TET2* was the most frequently mutated gene, occurring in 32% of the samples (10/31). NGS revealed nonsense mutations accompanied by the loss of heterozygosity in *TET2* and *MLL3*, suggesting important consequences of *MLL3* and *TET2* inactivation in the leukemogenesis of HTLV-1-induced ATL.

## 6.5 Epigenetic Abnormalities

### 6.5.1 DNA Methylation Abnormalities

The first report on DNA methylation of cellular genes was that of the *CDKN2* family. The *CDKN2* locus encodes proteins such as p16, p14, and p15 and is involved in cell cycle regulation and considered to be a hot spot of genomic and epigenomic abnormalities. Our copy number variation (CNV) analyses revealed the clustering of genomic deletions at this locus in 46 out of 168 cases (27%) [46]. Nosaka et al. conducted CpG methylation analyses, which showed DNA hypermethylation of this locus in 47% and 73% of acute-type and lymphoma-type ATL cases, respectively, whereas the methylation levels were 17% in both chronic- and smoldering-type ATL cases. Control samples from asymptomatic carriers and uninfected healthy volunteers did not reveal any methylation of this locus [85]. Hofman et al. reported that the levels of CpG methylation of *CDK2B* were higher than those of *CDK2A* [86].

A recent report described the progressive accumulation of CpG methylations of *HCAD*, *SHP1*, *DAPK*, and other genes in association with disease progression [79]. However, our expression profiling data of ATL samples did not show any downregulation in the expression of *CDKN2* family members. This underscores the importance of detailed analyses of expression levels and functional consequences of these cell cycle regulators in ATL cells [46]. *CDKN1A* ($p21^{waf/Cip1}$) has been reported to be downregulated by DNA methylation [73], which is in line with our data (46). These results suggest a relation between abnormal DNA methylation and cell cycle regulation and the possible breakdown of their functions.

DNA methylation analyses have also been reported for genes other than cell cycle regulators. In one study, high levels of DNA methylation of bone morphogenetic protein-6 (*BMP6*) were found in all subtypes of ATL, with higher levels in aggressive subtypes [87]. In one ATL patient, *BMP6* methylation was associated with progression from chronic to acute type, suggesting the functional involvement of this gene in tumor progression. DNA methylation of adenomatous polyposis coli (*APC*) has also been reported, suggesting that the downregulation of tumor suppressors may be involved in leukemogenesis and/or progression of ATL [88]. The downregulation of *CD26* expression has been found in ATL cells and has been documented as leading to the discrimination of these cells from normal T cells [89]. DNA methylation was shown to be involved in this downregulation [89]. Yasunaga et al. conducted a screening study using methylated CpG island amplification/representational difference analysis (MCA/RDA) of ATL cells [90]. They found abnormal DNA methylation in 53 genes, including those involved in apoptosis resistance such as *KLF4* and *EGR3*. They also reported the aberrant expression of *MEL1S*, an alternatively spliced variant of *MEL1* resulting from its hypomethylation, in ATL cells [91].

These data collectively suggest that changes in DNA methylation patterns are one of the molecular characteristics of ATL cells that contribute to their unique cellular phenotypes. A comprehensive description was not available until the completion of genetic and epigenetic landscape studies conducted by Ogawa and colleagues [67].

### 6.5.2 Abnormalities of Histone Modifications

Various chemical histone modifications are known to be involved in the modulation of the structure of chromatin and gene expression. Thus, complex aberrations of histone modifications are predicted in ATL cells, which constitute one rationale for profiling aberrant gene expression. However, mainly due to technical difficulties, significant progress has not been made in characterizing histone modifications in ATL cells, in contrast to an extensive number of DNA methylation studies.

Previous studies have provided firm evidence on the abnormalities of histone deacetylases (HDACs) in human tumor cells and their involvement in malignancy phenotypes. HDAC inhibitors play important roles in epigenetic studies. Specifically related to HTLV-1 and ATL, Nishioka et al. reported that HDAC inhibition induced apoptosis of HTLV-1-infected cell lines [92] and suppressed the constitutively active NF-κB pathway. In contrast, HDAC inhibitors have been shown to activate the NF-κB pathway by inducing RelA acetylation [93]. Thus, the effects of HDAC inhibitors on HTLV-1-infected cells remain contradictory and should be studied in detail. Genes with CpG islands are frequently regulated by the cooperative function of DNA methylation and histone acetylation. One example is *TBP-2*, which was downregulated by DNA methylation and histone deacetylation during the transformation of HTLV-1-infected T cells [94, 95]. Since *TBP-2* suppresses the proliferation of HTLV-1 infected T cells, it is conceivable that epigenetic deregulation of gene expression is directly involved in the regulation of ATL cell proliferation. Another report showed that a new HDAC inhibitor, AR42, successfully suppressed tumor cell growth in a mouse xenograft model of ATL [96]. The results of clinical trials with new HDAC inhibitors are expected.

In oncological research, methylation of histone 3 lysine 27 (H3K27) and its function have been extensively studied. The trimethylation of H3K27 (H3K28m3) is well known to be involved in the survival, proliferation, dedifferentiation, invasion, and metastasis of many human cancers, such as breast cancer and prostate cancer, as well as in B-cell lymphoma [97]. H3K27m3 is a marker for the suppression of gene expression in the euchromatin region. Polycomb group (PcG) proteins form multi-protein complexes that function as transcriptional repressors of several thousand genes controlling differentiation pathways during development. Although the mechanism by which PcG proteins work as transcriptional repressors is not completely understood, it is widely predicted to involve posttranslational chemical modifications of histones by two major PcG protein complexes: polycomb repressive complex 1 (PRC1) and polycomb repressive complex 2 (PRC2).

Fujikawa et al. recently conducted a comprehensive study on the polycomb-dependent epigenetic landscape of ATL cells to decipher the ATL-specific

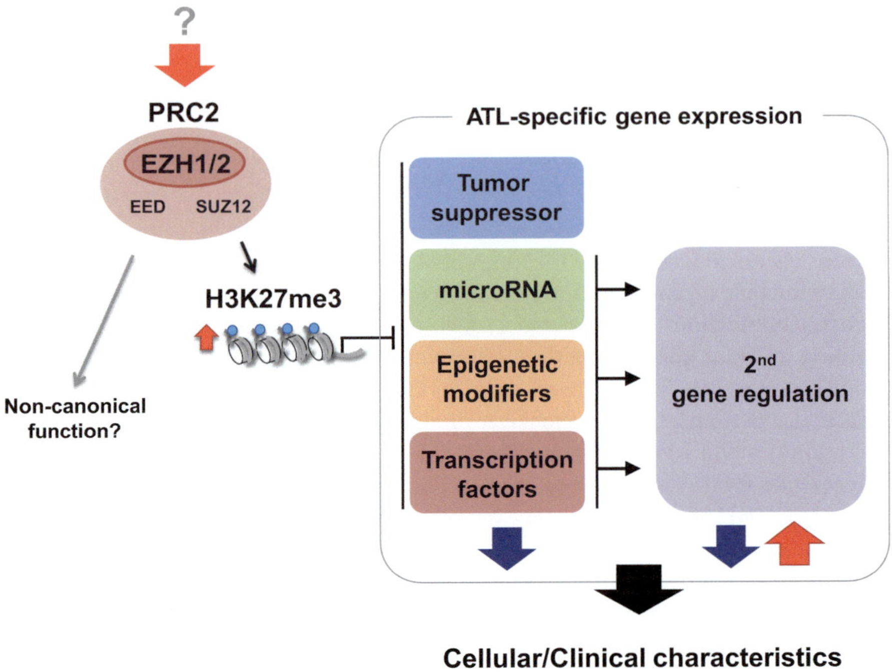


**Fig. 6.3** Epigenetic landscape of ATL. The predominant characteristic feature of an ATL epigenome is the accumulation of H3K27m3, which suppresses the expression of genes with important cellular functions. Downregulation of transcription factors, epigenetic modifiers, and miRNAs leads to secondary effects in gene regulation that determine cellular functions and clinical manifestations

epigenetic code critical for ATL pathogenesis [98]. Integrative analyses of the epigenome ($n = 3$) and transcriptome ($n = 58$) of primary ATL cells and corresponding normal $CD4^+$ T cells revealed that H3K27me3 was significantly and frequently reprogrammed in over half of the genes (53.8%) in ATL cells and that its pattern was distinct from other cancer types and PcG-dependent cell lineages. Downregulation of gene expression was associated with disease progression, which included key genes such as *miR-31*, *BCL2L11*, *EVC1/2*, *CDKN1A*, and *NDRG2*. Diverse outcomes were also found by the remote regulation of a broad spectrum of gene regulators, including various transcription factors, miRNAs, epigenetic modifiers, and developmental genes. The mutation of *EZH2* was not found in 50 ATL patients studied. High levels of EZH1 expression were confirmed in peripheral T cells, which compensated for the functions of *EZH2*. Thus, the simultaneous depletion of two H3K27me3 writers, EZH1 and EZH2, significantly diminished cellular H3K27me3 levels and dramatically inhibited ATL cell growth in comparison to single depletion, suggesting that the compensatory actions of EZH1/2 might be critical for ATL (Fig. 6.3).

## 6.6 Conclusion

Significant progress has been made in the field of ATL research. This research has provided extensive information on the cellular and molecular characteristics of ATL cells. However, several questions remain unanswered. First, information on the process of immortalization after HTLV-1 infection of T cells is limited due to the technical difficulties of in vitro infection experiments and the lack of appropriate animal models with HTLV-1 infection. Second, molecular events during clonal progression have not yet been well delineated. Because the reported landscape of genetic and epigenetic abnormalities is that of terminally transformed ATL cells, studies on HTLV-1-infected clones in various carrier states will provide crucial data on the mechanisms of immortalization and clonal expansion. Finally, there is insufficient information on the discrimination between low-risk and high-risk HTLV-1 carriers, although proviral load, one of the major risk factors, is evidently determined by host factors. Taken together, studies anticipated to delineate molecular processes involved in the natural history of HTLV-1 infection will provide the basis for the prevention and treatment of HTLV-1-associated diseases, including ATL.

## References

1. Uchiyama T, Yodoi J, Sagawa K, Takatsuki K, Uchino H. Adult T-cell leukemia: clinical and hematologic features of 16 cases. Blood. 1997;50:481–92.
2. Poiesz BJ, Ruscetti FW, Gazdar AF, Bunn PA, Minna JD, Gallo RC. Detection and isolation of type C retrovirus particles from fresh and cultured lymphocytes of a patient with cutaneous T-cell lymphoma. Proc Natl Acad Sci U S A. 1980;77:7415–9.
3. Shimoyama M. Diagnostic criteria and classification of clinical subtypes of adult T-cell leukaemia-lymphoma. A report from the Lymphoma Study Group (1984–87). Br J Haematol. 1991;79:428–39.
4. Okamoto T, Ohno Y, Tsugane S, et al. Multi-step carcinogenesis model for adult T-cell leukemia. Jpn J Cancer Res. 1989;80:191–5.
5. Yoshida M, Seiki M, Yamaguchi K, Takatsuki K. Monoclonal integration of human T-cell leukemia provirus in all primary tumors of adult T-cell leukemia suggests causative role of human T-cell leukemia virus in the disease. Proc Natl Acad Sci U S A. 1984;81:2534–7.
6. Yamaguchi K, Seiki M, Yoshida M, Nishimura H, Kawano F, Takatsuki K. The detection of human T cell leukemia virus proviral DNA and its application for classification and diagnosis of T cell malignancy. Blood. 1984;63:1235–40.
7. Kondo S, Kotani T, Tsumori S, et al. Identification of biclonal (duplex) leukemia cells expressing CD4+/CD8- or CD4−/CD8+ from a patient with adult T-cell leukemia/lymphoma. Br J Haematol. 1995;89:669–71.
8. Shibata K, Shimamoto Y, Suga K, et al. Adult T-cell leukemia/lymphoma with two distinct clones in peripheral blood and lymph node. Am J Hematol. 1995;48:116–9.
9. Shimamoto Y, Kikuchi M, Funai N, Suga K, Matsuzaki M, Yamaguchi M. Spontaneous remission in adult T-cell leukemia/lymphoma. Cancer. 1993;72:735–40.

10. Kato N, Sugawara H, Aoyagi S, Mayuzumi M. Lymphoma-type adult T-cell leukemia-lymphoma with a bulky cutaneous tumor showing multiple human T-lymphotropic virus-1 DNA integration. Br J Haematol. 2001;144:1244–8.
11. Tsukasaki K, Tsushima H, Yamamura M, et al. Integration patterns of HTLV-1 provirus in relation to the clinical course of ATL: frequent clonal change at crisis from indolent disease. Blood. 1997;89:948–56.
12. Umino A, Nakagawa M, Utsunomiya A, Tsukasaki K, Taira N, Katayama N, Seto M. Clonal evolution of adult T-cell leukemia/lymphoma takes place in the lymph nodes. Blood. 2011;117:5473–8. doi:10.1182/blood-2010-12-327791.
13. Umino A, Seto M. Array CGH reveals clonal evolution of adult T-cell leukemia/lymphoma. Methods Mol Biol. 2013;973:189–96. doi:10.1007/978-1-62703-281-0_12.
14. Takemoto S, Matsuoka M, Yamaguchi K, Takatsuki K. A novel diagnostic method of adult T-cell leukemia: monoclonal integration of human T-cell lymphotropic virus type I provirus DNA detected by inverse polymerase chain reaction. Blood. 1994;84:3080–5.
15. Etoh K, Tamiya S, Yamaguchi K, Okayama A, Tsubouchi H, Ideta T, Mueller N, Takatsuki K, Matsuoka M. Persistent clonal proliferation of human T-lymphotropic virus type I-infected cells in vivo. Cancer Res. 1997;57:4862–7.
16. Ohshima K, Mukai Y, Shiraki H, Suzumiya J, Tashiro K, Kikuchi M. Clonal integration and expression of human T-cell lymphotropic virus type I in carriers detected by polymerase chain reaction and inverse PCR. Am J Hematol. 1997;54:306–12.
17. Eiraku N, Hingorani R, Ijichi S, et al. Clonal expansion within CD4+ and CD8+ T cell subsets in human T lymphotropic virus type I-infected individuals. J Immunol. 1998;161:6674–80.
18. Okayama A, Stuver S, Iga M, et al. Sequential change of virus markers in seroconverters with community-acquired infection of human T lymphotropic virus type I. J Infect Dis. 2001;183:1031–107.
19. Tanaka G, Okayama A, Watanabe T, et al. The clonal expansion of human T lymphotropic virus type 1-infected T cells: a comparison between seroconverters and long-term carriers. J Infect Dis. 2005;191:1140–7.
20. Cavrois M, Wain-Hobson S, Wattel E. Stochastic events in the amplification of HTLV-I integration sites by linker-mediated PCR. Res Virol. 1995;146:179–84.
21. Cavrois M, Gessain A, Wain-Hobson S, Wattel E. Proliferation of HTLV-1 infected circulating cells in vivo in all asymptomatic carriers and patients with TSP/HAM. Oncogene. 1996;12:2419–23.
22. Gabet AS, Mortreux F, Talarmin A, et al. High circulating proviral load with oligoclonal expansion of HTLV-1 bearing T cells in HTLV-1 carriers with strongyloidiasis. Oncogene. 2000;19:4954–60.
23. Gillet NA, Malani N, Melamed A, et al. The host genomic environment of the provirus determines the abundance of HTLV-1-infected T-cell clones. Blood. 2011;117:3113–22. doi:10.1182/blood-2010-10-312926.
24. Melamed A, Laydon DJ, Gillet NA, Tanaka Y, Taylor GP, Bangham CR. Genome-wide determinants of proviral targeting, clonal abundance and expression in natural HTLV-1 infection. PLoS Pathog. 2013;9:e1003271. doi:10.1371/journal.ppat.1003271.
25. Cook LB, Melamed A, Niederer H, et al. The role of HTLV-1 clonality, proviral structure, and genomic integration site in adult T-cell leukemia/lymphoma. Blood. 2014;123:3925–31. doi:10.1182/blood-2014-02-553602.
26. Firouzi S, López Y, Suzuki Y, Nakai K, Sugano S, Yamochi T, Watanabe T. Development and validation of a new high-throughput method to investigate the clonality of HTLV-1-infected cells based on provirus integration sites. Genome Med. 2014;6:46. doi:10.1186/gm568. eCollection 2014
27. Kobayashi S, Nakano K, Watanabe E, et al. CADM1 expression and stepwise downregulation of CD7 are closely associated with clonal expansion of HTLV-1-infected cells in adult T-cell leukemia/lymphoma. Clin Cancer Res. 2014;20:2851–61. doi:10.1158/1078-0432.CCR-13-3169.

28. Kobayashi S, Watanabe E, Ishigaki T, et al. Advanced HTLV-1 carriers and early-stage indolent ATLs are indistinguishable based on CADM1 positivity in flow cytometry. Cancer Sci. 2015;106:598–603. doi:10.1111/cas.12639.
29. Rosenblatt JD, Miles S, Gasson JC, Prager D. Transactivation of cellular genes by human retroviruses. Curr Top Microbiol Immunol. 1995;193:25–49.
30. Bertini R, Luini W, Sozzani S, et al. Identification of MIP-1 alpha/LD78 as a monocyte chemoattractant released by the HTLV-1-transformed cell line MT-4. AIDS Res Hum Retrovir. 1995;11:155–60.
31. Baba M, Imai T, Yoshida T, Yoshie O. Constitutive expression of various chemokine genes in human T-cell lines infected with human T-cell leukemia virus type 1: role of the viral transactivator Tax. Int J Cancer. 1996;66:124–9.
32. Hasegawa H, Nomura T, Kohno M, et al. Increased chemokine receptor CCR7/EBI1 expression enhances the infiltration of lymphoid organs by adult T-cell leukemia cells. Blood. 2000;95:30–8.
33. Yoshie O, Fujisawa R, Nakayama T, et al. Frequent expression of CCR4 in adult T-cell leukemia and human T-cell leukemia virus type 1-transformed T cells. Blood. 2002;99:1505–11.
34. Kuramochi M, Fukuhara H, Nobukuni T, et al. TSLC1 is a tumor-suppressor gene in human non-small-cell lung cancer. Nat Genet. 2001;27:427–30.
35. Sasaki H, Nishikata I, Shiraga T, et al. Overexpression of a cell adhesion molecule, TSLC1, as a possible molecular marker for acute-type adult T-cell leukemia. Blood. 2005;105:1204–13.
36. Watanabe T, Yamaguchi K, Takatsuki K, Osame M, Yoshida M. Constitutive expression of parathyroid hormone-related protein gene in human T cell leukemia virus type 1 (HTLV-1) carriers and adult T cell leukemia patients that can be trans-activated by HTLV-1 tax gene. J Exp Med. 1990;172:759–65.
37. Ishikawa T, Imura A, Tanaka K, et al. E-selectin and vascular cell adhesion molecule-1 mediate adult T-cell leukemia cell adhesion to endothelial cells. Blood. 1992;82:1590–8.
38. Imura A, Hori T, Imada K, et al. The human OX40/gp34 system directly mediates adhesion of activated T cells to vascular endothelial cells. J Exp Med. 1996;183:2185–95.
39. Tatewaki M, Yamaguchi K, Matsuoka M, et al. Constitutive overexpression of the L-selectin gene in fresh leukemic cells of adult T-cell leukemia that can be transactivated by human T-cell lymphotropic virus type 1 Tax. Blood. 1995;86:3109–17.
40. Uchiyama T, Ishikawa T, Imura A. Cell adhesion molecules in HTLV-I infection. J AIDS Hum Retrovirol. 1996;13(Suppl 1):S114–8.
41. Koizumi S, Iwanaga M, Imai S, et al. Expression of myeloid cell phenotypes by a novel adult T-cell leukemia/lymphoma cell line. J Natl Cancer Inst. 1992;84:690–3.
42. Tricarico M, Macchi B, D'Atri S, Morrone S, Bonmassar E, Fuggetta MP, Graziani G. In vitro infection of CD4+ T lymphocytes with HTLV-1 generates immortalized cell lines coexpressing lymphoid and myeloid cell markers. Leukemia. 1999;13:222–9.
43. Pichler K, Schneider G, Grassmann R. Microrna mir-146a and further oncogenesis-related cellular micrornas are dysregulated in HTLV-1-transformed T lymphocytes. Retrovirology. 2008;5:e100.
44. Bellon M, Lepelletier Y, Hermine O, Nicot C. Deregulation of microrna involved in hematopoiesis and the immune response in HTLV-I adult T-cell leukemia. Blood. 2009;113:4914–7.
45. Yeung ML, Yasunaga J, Bennasser Y, et al. Roles for micrornas, miR-93 and miR-130b, and tumor protein 53-induced nuclear protein 1 tumor suppressor in cell growth dysregulation by human T-cell lymphotrophic virus 1. Cancer Res. 2008;68:8976–85.
46. Yamagishi M, Nakano K, Miyake A, et al. Polycomb-mediated loss of miR-31 activates nik-dependent NF- κb pathway in adult T cell leukemia and other cancers. Cancer Cell. 2012;21:121–35.
47. Mori N, Fujii M, Ikeda S, Yamada Y, Tomonaga M, Ballard DW, Yamamoto N. Constitutive activation of NF-kappaB in primary adult T-cell leukemia cells. Blood. 1999;93:2360–8.

48. Watanabe M, Ohsugi T, Shoda M, et al. Dual targeting of transformed and untransformed HTLV-1-infected T cells by DHMEQ, a potent and selective inhibitor of NF-kappaB, as a strategy for chemoprevention and therapy of adult T-cell leukemia. Blood. 2005;106:2462–71.
49. Fukuda R, Hayashi A, Utsunomiya A, et al. Alteration of phosphatidylinositol 3-kinase cascade in the multilobulated nuclear formation of adult T cell leukemia/lymphoma (ATLL). Proc Natl Acad Sci U S A. 2005;102:15213–8.
50. Takemoto S, Mulloy JC, Cereseto A, et al. Proliferation of adult T cell leukemia/lymphoma cells is associated with the constitutive activation of JAK/STAT proteins. Proc Natl Acad Sci U S A. 1997;94:13897–902.
51. Kamada N, Sakurai M, Miyamoto K, et al. Chromosome abnormalities in adult T-cell leukemia/lymphoma: a karyotype review committee report. Cancer Res. 1992;52:1481–93.
52. Itoyama T, Chaganti RS, Yamada Y, et al. Cytogenetic analysis and clinical significance in adult T-cell leukemia/lymphoma: a study of 50 cases from the human T-cell leukemia virus type-1 endemic area, Nagasaki. Blood. 2001;97:3612–20.
53. Tsukasaki K, Krebs J, Nagai K, Tomonaga M, Koeffler HP, Bartram CR, Jauch A. Comparative genomic hybridization analysis in adult T-cell leukemia/lymphoma: correlation with clinical course. Blood. 2001;97:3875–81.
54. Sakashita A, Hattori T, Miller CW, et al. Mutations of the p53 gene in adult T-cell leukemia. Blood. 1992;79:477–80.
55. Cesarman E, Chadburn A, Inghirami G, Gaidano G, Knowles DM. Structural and functional analysis of oncogenes and tumor suppressor genes in adult T-cell leukemia/lymphoma shows frequent p53 mutations. Blood. 1992;80:3205–16.
56. Nagai H, Kinoshita T, Imamura J, et al. Genetic alteration of p53 in some patients with adult T-cell leukemia. Jpn J Cancer Res. 1991;82:1421–7.
57. Tawara M, Hogerzeil SJ, Yamada Y, et al. Impact of p53 aberration on the progression of adult T-cell leukemia/lymphoma. Cancer Lett. 2006;234:249–55.
58. Gaidano G, Ballerini P, Gong JZ, et al. p53 mutations in human lymphoid malignancies: association with Burkitt lymphoma and chronic lymphocytic leukemia. Proc Natl Acad Sci U S A. 1991;88:5413–7.
59. Yamato K, Oka T, Hiroi M, et al. Aberrant expression of the p53 tumor suppressor gene in adult T-cell leukemia and HTLV- I-infected cells. Jpn J Cancer Res. 1993;84:4–8.
60. Reid RL, Lindholm PF, Mireskandari A, Dittmer J, Brady JN. Stabilization of wild-type p53 in human T-lymphocytes transformed by HTLV-I. Oncogene. 1993;8:3029–36.
61. Takemoto S, Trovato R, Cereseto A, et al. p53 Stabilization and functional impairment in the absence of genetic mutation or the alteration of the p14(APF)-MDM2 loop in ex vivo and cultured adult T-cell leukemia/lymphoma cells. Blood. 2000;95:3939–44.
62. Akagi T, Ono H, Tsuchida N, Shimotohno K. Aberrant expression and function of p53 in T cells immortalized by HTLV-I Tax1. FEBS Lett. 1997;406:263–6.
63. Pise-Masison CA, Choi K-S, Radonovich M, Dittmer J, Kim S-J, Brady JN. Inhibition of p53 transactivation function by the human T-cell lymphotropic virus type 1 Tax protein. J Virol. 1998;72:1165–70.
64. Pise-Masison CA, Mahieux R, Jiang H, et al. Inactivation of p53 by human T-cell lymphotropic virus type 1 tax requires activation of the NF-κB pathway and is dependent on p53 phosphorylation. Mol Cell Biol. 2000;20:3377–86.
65. Mulloy JC, Kislyakova T, Cereseto A, et al. Human T-cell lymphotropic/leukemia virus type 1 tax abrogates p53-induced cell cycle arrest and apoptosis through its CREB/ATF functional domain. J Virol. 1998;72:8852–60.
66. Pise-Masison CA, Mahieux R, Radonovich M, Jiang H, Brady JN. Human T-lymphotropic virus type I Tax protein utilizes distinct pathways for p53 inhibition that are cell type-dependent. J Biol Chem. 2001;276:200–5.
67. Kataoka K, Nagata Y, Kitanaka A, et al. Integrated molecular analysis of adult T cell leukemia/lymphoma. Nat Genet. 2015;47:1304–15. doi:10.1038/ng.3415.
68. Sherr CJ. Principles of tumor suppression. Cell. 2004;116:235–46.

69. Williams RT, Sherr CJ. The INK4-ARF (CDKN2A/B) locus in hematopoiesis and BCR-ABL -induced leukemias. Cold Spring Harb Symp Quant Biol. 2008;73:461–7.
70. Trovato R, Cereseto A, Takemoto S, et al. Deletion of the p164*A* gene in ex vivo acute adult T cell lymphoma/leukemia cells and methylation of the p164*A* promoter in HTLV type I-infected T cell lines. AIDS Res Hum Retrovir. 2000;16:709–13.
71. Uchida T, Kinoshita T, Murate T, Saito H, Hotta T. CDKN2 (MTS1/p164) gene alterations in adult T-cell leukemia/lymphoma. Leuk Lymphoma. 1998;29:27–35.
72. Hatta Y, Hirama T, Miller CW, Yamada Y, Tomonaga M, Koeffler HP. Homozygous deletions of the p15 (MTS2) and p16 (CDKN2/MTS1) genes in adult T-cell leukemia. Blood. 1995;85:2699–704.
73. Watanabe M, Nakahata S, Hamasaki M, et al. Downregulation of CDKN1A in adult T-cell leukemia/lymphoma despite overexpression of CDKN1A in human T-lymphotropic virus 1-infected cell lines. J Virol. 2010;84:6966–77.
74. Hatta Y, Yamada Y, Tomonaga M, Koeffler HP. Extensive analysis of the retinoblastoma gene in adult T cell leukemia/lymphoma (ATL). Leukemia. 1997;11:984–9.
75. Takeuchi S, Takeuchi N, Tsukasaki K, et al. Mutations in the retinoblastoma-related gene RB2/p130 in adult T-cell leukaemia/lymphoma. Leuk Lymphoma. 2003;44:699–701.
76. Hangaishi A, Ogawa S, Imamura N, et al. Inactivation of multiple tumor-suppressor genes involved in negative regulation of the cell cycle, MTS1/p16INK4A/CDKN2, MTS2/p15INK4B, p53, and Rb genes in primary lymphoid malignancies. Blood. 1996;87:4949–58.
77. Nakayama K, Yamada Y, Koji T, Hayashi T, Tomonaga M, Kamihira S. Expression and phosphorylation status of retinoblastoma protein in adult T-cell leukemia/lymphoma. Leuk Res. 2000;24:299–305.
78. Krystal G, Damen JE, Helgason CD, et al. SHIPs ahoy. Int J Biochem Cell Biol. 1999;31:1007–10.
79. Sato H, Oka T, Shinnou Y, et al. Multi-step aberrant CpG island hyper-methylation is associated with the progression of adult T-cell leukemia/lymphoma. Am J Pathol. 2010;176:402–15.
80. Nakahata S, Morishita K. CADM1/TSLC1 is a novel cell surface marker for adult T-cell leukemia/lymphoma. J Clin Exp Hematopathol. 2012;52(1):17–22.
81. Asanuma S, Yamagishi M, Kawanami K, et al. Adult T-cell leukemia cells are characterized by abnormalities of Helios expression that promotes T-cell growth. Cancer Sci. 2013;104:1097–106. doi:10.1111/cas.12181.
82. Kataoka K, Shiraishi Y, Takeda Y, et al. Aberrant PD-L1 expression through 3′-UTR disruption in multiple cancers. Nature. 2016; doi:10.1038/nature18294.
83. Nagata Y, Kontani K, Enami T, et al. Variegated RHOA mutations in adult T-cell leukemia/lymphoma. Blood. 2016;127:596–604. doi:10.1182/blood-2015-06-644948.
84. Yeh CH, Bai XT, Moles R, Ratner L, Waldmann TA, Watanabe T, Nicot C. Mutation of epigenetic regulators TET2 and MLL3 in patients with HTLV-I-induced acute adult T-cell leukemia. Mol Cancer. 2016;15:15. doi:10.1186/s12943-016-0500-z.
85. Nosaka K, Maeda M, Tamiya S, et al. Increasing methylation of the CDKN2A gene is associated with the progression of adult T-cell leukemia. Cancer Res. 2000;60:1043–8.
86. Hofmann WK, Tsukasaki K, Takeuchi N, et al. Methylation analysis of cell cycle control genes in adult T-cell leukemia/lymphoma. Leuk Lymphoma. 2001;42:1107–9.
87. Taniguchi A, Nemoto Y, Yokoyama A, Kotani N, Imai S, Shuin T, Daibata M. Promoter methylation of the bone morphogenetic protein-6 gene in association with adult T-cell leukemia. Int J Cancer. 2008;123:1824–31. doi:10.1002/ijc.23749.
88. Yang Y, Takeuchi S, Tsukasaki K, et al. Methylation analysis of the adenomatous polyposis coli (APC) gene in adult T-cell leukemia/lymphoma. Leuk Res. 2005;29:47–51.
89. Tsuji T, Sugahara K, Tsuruda K, et al. Clinical and oncologic implications in epigenetic downregulation of CD26/dipeptidyl peptidase IV in adult T-cell leukemia cells. Int J Hematol. 2004;80:254–60.

90. Yasunaga J, Taniguchi Y, Nosaka K, et al. Identification of aberrantly methylated genes in association with adult T-cell leukemia. Cancer Res. 2004;64:6002–9.
91. Yoshida M, Nosaka K, Yasunaga J, et al. Aberrant expression of the MEL1S gene identified in association with hypomethylation in adult T-cell leukemia cells. Blood. 2004;103:2753–60.
92. Nishioka C, Ikezoe T, Yang J, et al. Histone deacetylase inhibitors induce growth arrest and apoptosis of HTLV-1-infected T-cells via blockade of signaling by nuclear factor kappa B. Leuk Res. 2008;32:287–96.
93. Chiechio S, Zammataro M, Morales ME, et al. Epigenetic modulation of mGlu2 receptors by histone deacetylase inhibitors in the treatment of inflammatory pain. Mol Pharmacol. 2009;75:1014–20.
94. Ahsan MK, Masutani H, Yamaguchi Y, et al. Loss of interleukin-2-dependency in HTLV-I -infected T cells on gene silencing of thioredoxin-binding protein-2. Oncogene. 2006;25:2181–91.
95. Nishinaka Y, Nishiyama A, Masutani H, et al. Loss of thioredoxin-binding protein-2/vitamin D3 up-regulated protein 1 in human T-cell leukemia virus type I-dependent T-cell transformation: implications for adult T-cell leukemia leukemogenesis. Cancer Res. 2004;64:1287–92.
96. Zimmerman B, Sargeant A, Landes K, Fernandez SA, Chen CS, Lairmore MD. Efficacy of novel histone deacetylase inhibitor, AR42, in a mouse model of, human T-lymphotropic virus type 1 adult T cell lymphoma. Leuk Res. 2011;35:1491–7.
97. Sparmann A, van Lohuizen M. Polycomb silencers control cell fate, development and cancer. Nat Rev Cancer. 2006;6:846–56.
98. Fujikawa D, Nakagawa S, Hori M, et al. Polycomb-dependent epigenetic landscape in adult T-cell leukemia. Blood. 2016;127:1790–802. doi:10.1182/blood-2015-08-662593.

# Chapter 7
# Clinical Features of Adult T-cell Leukemia/ Lymphoma (ATL)

**Yoshitaka Imaizumi**

## 7.1 Clinical Features of Adult T-cell leukemia-lymphoma (ATL)

Adult T-cell leukemia-lymphoma (ATL) is a distinct T-cell malignancy caused by human T-cell leukemia virus type I (HTLV-1) [15, 20]. ATL usually develops in elderly carriers of HTLV-1, and recent analysis has shown that the median age of ATL patients is increasing. Serial nationwide surveys of ATL patients have clearly demonstrated this trend. The mean age of ATL patients has gradually increased from 52.7 years in the first survey (cases before 1980) to 61.1 years in the ninth survey (1996–1997) and finally to 66.0 years in the most recent survey (2006–2007) (The T- and B-cell Malignancy Study Group. 1981, [18]).

ATL is known as "leukemic lymphoma" and has an extremely poor prognosis [15]. However, its onset and clinical course are highly heterogeneous among patients [4]. In some patients, inspection-level abnormalities such as leukocytosis and abnormal lymphocytes in the peripheral blood (PB) are present without any symptoms and eventually lead to the diagnosis of ATL. Some patients visit a dermatologist with skin lesions that are the only clinical symptom. In contrast, some patients present with high fever, disturbance of consciousness, and organ failure. Because the general condition of these patients has already become very poor at the time of consultation, they have a very aggressive clinical course.

The involvement of multiple extranodal lesions is an important clinical feature of ATL [5]. ATL is a malignancy of mature lymphocytes, and thus, lymphadenopathy is frequently observed among ATL patients. However, many ATL patients also experience extranodal lesions in sites such as the PB, skin, lung, gastrointestinal tract, bone, central nervous system, ascites, and pleural effusion, among others. The

Y. Imaizumi (✉)
Department of Hematology, Nagasaki University Hospital, Nagasaki, Japan
e-mail: y-imaizm@nagasaki-u.ac.jp



T. Watanabe, T. Fukushima (eds.), *Adult T-cell Leukemia/Lymphoma*,
DOI 10.1007/978-4-431-56523-9_7

combination of extranodal lesions and the various degrees of involvement generate highly heterogeneous clinical features in ATL. The leukemic manifestation is one of the most distinctive features of ATL. The abnormal cells in PB are typically multi-lobulated and have condensed nuclei with basophilic cytoplasm. Such cells are called "flower cells" and are the characteristic morphology of ATL [10]. The skin is also frequently involved in ATL. Several types of skin lesions have been reported in ATL, and a relationship between the type of skin lesion and the prognosis of ATL has also been shown [9]. Thus, careful observation of not only the presence of skin lesions but also the type is important for clinicians. ATL cells invade multiple organs, and therefore, ATL patients often have a high tumor burden in addition to complications such as the dysfunction of organs including the liver and/or kidney [17]. A high number of involved lesions and tumor burden are poor prognostic factors [5].

Infection is an important complication of ATL [11]. Infections are present in 26% of ATL patients at the initial presentation, and more than half are fungal or viral infections. In ATL patients, CD4-positive T cells are infected with HTLV-1 and have transformed into malignant cells; thus, the normal function of CD4-positive T cells is lost. Suppressed or altered function has been reported in HTLV-1-infected T cells [7, 16]. Thus, cellular immunity is severely impaired, resulting in frequent opportunistic infections such as cytomegalovirus infection, pneumocystis pneumonia, fungus infection, and strongyloidiasis, among others [11]. Bacterial infections such as bacterial pneumonia and bacteremia also occur frequently during the course of the disease. In some patients, severe infections become the main cause of death [11]. Thus, the diagnosis and treatment of infectious complications are very important in the clinical management of ATL.

Hypercalcemia, another important complication of ATL, causes nausea, vomiting, constipation, thirst, frequent urination, and a disturbance in consciousness. Renal dysfunction may occur in severe cases [11]. Several factors such as parathyroid hormone-related peptide and the receptor activator of nuclear factor-kappa B ligand are involved in hypercalcemia in ATL [2, 6].

These complications (opportunistic infection and hypercalcemia) and a large tumor burden result in a poor general condition and performance status. These factors are correlated with difficulties in the treatment of ATL. For such patients, modification of the dose of anticancer agents and adequate supportive care for severe complications are necessary.

## 7.2 Diagnosis of ATL

In practice, the diagnosis of ATL is made clinically when a patient with peripheral T-cell lymphoma (PTCL) is anti-HTLV-1 antibody positive [11]. In many patients with ATL, abnormal lymphocytes (flower cells) appear in PB, but "atypical" abnormal lymphocytes (ATL cells), which are small with a mature nuclear texture and an incised or lobulated nucleus, are also seen in some patients. The analysis of cell surface antigens by flow cytometry is very useful for diagnosis. Typically, ATL cells show CD3-positive/dull, CD4-positive, CD8-negative, and CD25-positive phenotypes. However, ATL cells show aberrant phenotypes in some patients [3]. Recently, expression of CC chemokine receptor 4 (CCR4), a type of chemokine receptor, has been reported in most ATL cases [1, 19]. The expression of cell adhesion molecule 1/tumor suppressor in lung cancer 1 (CADM1/TSLC1) has also been reported [8]. These cell surface markers are expected to become useful markers for the detection of HTLV-1-infected ATL cells. The details of the immunophenotype of ATL cells are described in another chapter of this issue. When abnormal lymphocytes or lymphocytosis are not detected in PB, a biopsy of the involved lesion is required for the pathological diagnosis of ATL or PTCL. The monoclonal proliferation of HTLV-1-infected cells can be detected with Southern blot hybridization (SBH) analysis of PB and/or biopsied samples from ATL patients [21]. SBH analysis is a useful tool for distinguishing ATL from other types of PTCL in HTLV-1 carriers. However, when the number of tumor cells in the sample is not sufficient, a false negative may occur. We should remember the sensitivity of SBH analysis and the quantity of the specimen required for SBH.

## 7.3 Clinical Subtypes of ATL

Most ATL patients have abnormal cells in PB. Such patients are categorized as stage IV in the Ann Arbor staging classification, which has been widely utilized for staging patients with Hodgkin or non-Hodgkin lymphoma. Because of the leukemic nature of ATL, the Ann Arbor staging does not reflect the natural progression of ATL and is not always useful for determining the treatment strategy. According to the clinical manifestation and natural history, clinical subtypes of ATL were proposed and are useful for determining a prognosis. ATL is divided into four clinical subtypes: acute, lymphoma, chronic, and smoldering (Table 7.1) [11]. In a retrospective study of 818 ATL patients in Japan, the median survival time was 6.2 months for the acute type, 10.2 months for the lymphoma type, 24.3 months for the chronic type, and not yet reached for the smoldering type. Thus, clinical subtype classification should be determined to decide the treatment strategy for each patient.

### *7.3.1 Lymphoma Type*

Patients with histologically proven lymphadenopathy and no abnormal lymphocytes in PB ($<1\%$ and no lymphocytosis) are classified as the lymphoma type. The precise differential diagnosis of ATL and other PTCL in HTLV-1 carriers is sometimes difficult, especially for non-leukemic types such as the lymphoma type, without the result of HTLV-1 SBH analysis.

**Table 7.1** Diagnostic criteria for the clinical subtype of ATL

| | Smoldering | Chronic | Lymphoma | Acute |
|---|---|---|---|---|
| Anti-HTLV-1 antibody | + | + | + | + |
| Lymphocyte ($\times 10^3$/mm$^3$) | <4 | ≧4 | <4 | [a] |
| Abnormal lymphocyte | ≧5% | + | ≦1% | [a] |
| Flower cells | [a] | [a] | No | [a] |
| LDH | ≦1.5ULN | ≦2ULN | [a] | [a] |
| Corrected calcium | <5.5mEq/l | <5.5mEq/l | [a] | [a] |
| Histology-proven lymphadenopathy | No | [a] | Yes | [a] |
| Tumor lesion | – | – | – | – |
| Skin | [a] | [a] | [a] | [a] |
| Lung | [a] | [a] | [a] | [a] |
| Lymph node | No | [a] | Yes | [a] |
| Liver | No | [a] | [a] | [a] |
| Spleen | No | [a] | [a] | [a] |
| CNS | No | No | [a] | [a] |
| Bone | No | No | [a] | [a] |
| Ascites | No | No | [a] | [a] |
| Pleural effusion | No | No | [a] | [a] |
| GI tract | No | No | [a] | [a] |

Modified from Shimoyama [11]
Histologically proven tumor lesions are required, if abnormal lymphocytes in peripheral blood are less than 5% in the smoldering, chronic, and acute type
*ULN* upper limit of normal, *CNS* central nervous system, *GI tract* gastrointestinal tract
[a]No essential qualification except terms required for other subtypes

## *7.3.2 Chronic Type*

Patients with absolute lymphocytosis (≥4000/mm$^3$) and >5% morphologically abnormal lymphocytes in PB are classified as chronic ATL. If <5% abnormal lymphocytes are present in PB, histologically proven skin and/or pulmonary lesions are required for the diagnosis of chronic ATL. The serum lactate dehydrogenase (LDH) level should be less than twice the normal upper limit, and the serum calcium level should be normal (<5.5 mEq/l). Lymphadenopathy and some extranodal organ involvement such as the skin, lung, liver, and spleen are allowed as criteria for the chronic type. However, involvement of the central nervous system, bone, and gastrointestinal tract is not allowed. Ascites and pleural effusions are also not allowed for the chronic type. For patients with chronic ATL, three poor prognostic factors have been identified: decreased serum albumin, increased serum LDH, and increased blood urea nitrogen [12]. Chronic ATL patients with normal values for these three factors have a favorable prognosis and account for about 30% of chronic ATL.

### 7.3.3 Smoldering Type

Patients with a normal absolute lymphocyte count ($<4,000/mm^3$) and $\geq 5\%$ of abnormal lymphocytes in PB without lymphadenopathies are classified as the smoldering type. The LDH levels should be $<1.5$ times the upper limit, and serum calcium should be $<5.5$ mEq/l. Skin and/or pulmonary involvement of ATL cells is allowed as a criterion for smoldering ATL, although other extranodal organ lesions are not. If abnormal lymphocytes are $<5\%$ in PB, histologically proven skin and/or pulmonary lesions are required for the diagnosis of smoldering ATL.

### 7.3.4 Acute Type

ATL patients not considered having the smoldering, chronic, or lymphoma types are classified as having the acute type. Most acute-type ATL patients have abnormal lymphocytes in PB. However, patients without abnormal lymphocytes in PB should be classified as having the acute type only if they have extranodal lesions, except in the skin or lung, and have no lymphadenopathy; such patients may be rare.

### 7.3.5 Indolent and Aggressive ATL

These clinical subtypes are closely related to the prognosis and are used for stratification of the treatment of ATL patients. The smoldering type and the chronic type without any of the three poor prognostic factors are called indolent ATL. On the other hand, the chronic type with any of the poor prognostic factors, acute type, and lymphoma type are called aggressive ATL [14].

### 7.3.6 Points to Notice Regarding the Clinical Subtypes of ATL

Some indolent ATL patients progress to a more aggressive disease status, a situation that is called "crisis" [13]. In general, patients with progression from indolent to aggressive ATL are in a state of crisis and are candidates for systemic chemotherapy. However, we should note that no precise criterion for the diagnosis of "crisis" has been established. The criteria for the clinical subtype of ATL were originally made by using clinical data at the time of diagnosis of ATL. These criteria have not been validated for the management of patients with clinical progression including "crisis."

Another point is important for subtype classification. The borderline of these subtypes is not always clear. One problem is due to the fact that morphological detection of abnormal lymphocytes is sometimes difficult. For example, smoldering ATL patients without skin and/or pulmonary lesions and HTLV-1 carriers are distinguished according to the percentage of abnormal lymphocytes in PB. Thus, the differential diagnosis may be difficult if the number of abnormal lymphocytes in PB is small. A similar situation occurs for distinguishing lymphoma from acute types of ATL.

## References

1. Ishida T, Utsunomiya A, Iida S, Inagaki H, Takatsuka Y, Kusumoto S, Takeuchi G, Shimizu S, Ito M, Komatsu H, Wakita A, Eimoto T, Matsushima K, Ueda R. Clinical significance of CCR4 expression in adult T-cell leukemia/lymphoma: its close association with skin involvement and unfavorable outcome. Clin Cancer Res. 2003;9(10 Pt 1):3625–34.
2. Honda S, Yamaguchi K, Miyake Y, Hayashi N, Adachi N, Kinoshita K, Ikehara O, Kimura S, Kinoshita T, Shimotohno K, et al. Production of parathyroid hormone-related protein in adult T-cell leukemia cells. Jpn J Cancer Res. 1988;79(12):1264–8.
3. Kamihira S, Sohda H, Atogami S, Toriya K, Yamada Y, Tsukazaki K, Momita S, Ikeda S, Kusano M, Amagasaki T, et al. Phenotypic diversity and prognosis of adult T-cell leukemia. Leuk Res. 1992;16(5):435–41.
4. Kawano F, Yamaguchi K, Nishimura H, Tsuda H, Takatsuki K. Variation in the clinical courses of adult T-cell leukemia. Cancer. 1985;55(4):851–6.
5. Lymphoma Study Group (1984–1987). Major prognostic factors of patients with adult T-cell leukemia-lymphoma: a cooperative study. Leuk Res. 1991;15(2–3):81–90.
6. Nosaka K, Miyamoto T, Sakai T, Mitsuya H, Suda T, Matsuoka M. Mechanism of hypercalcemia in adult T-cell leukemia: overexpression of receptor activator of nuclear factor kappaB ligand on adult T-cell leukemia cells. Blood. 2002;99(2):634–40.
7. Popovic M, Flomenberg N, Volkman DJ, Mann D, Fauci AS, Dupont B, Gallo RC. Alteration of T-cell functions by infection with HTLV-I or HTLV-II. Science. 1984;226(4673):459–62.
8. Sasaki H, Nishikata I, Shiraga T, Akamatsu E, Fukami T, Hidaka T, Kubuki Y, Okayama A, Hamada K, Okabe H, Murakami Y, Tsubouchi H, Morishita K. Overexpression of a cell adhesion molecule, TSLC1, as a possible molecular marker for acute-type adult T-cell leukemia. Blood. 2005;105(3):1204–13.
9. Sawada Y, Hino R, Hama K, Ohmori S, Fueki H, Yamada S, Fukamachi S, Tajiri M, Kubo R, Yoshioka M, Nakashima D, Sugita K, Yoshiki R, Shimauchi T, Mori T, Izu K, Kobayashi M, Nakamura M, Tokura Y. Type of skin eruption is an independent prognostic indicator for adult T-cell leukemia/lymphoma. Blood. 2011;117(15):3961–7.
10. Shimoyama M, Minato K, Tobinai K, Nagai M, Setoya T, Takenaka T, Ishihara K, Watanabe S, Hoshino H, Miwa M, Kinoshita M, Okabe S, Fukushima N, Inada N. Atypical adult T-cell leukemia-lymphoma: diverse clinical manifestations of adult T-cell leukemia-lymphoma. Jpn J Clin Oncol. 1983;13(Suppl 2):165–87.
11. Shimoyama M. Diagnostic criteria and classification of clinical subtypes of adult T-cell leukaemia-lymphoma. A report from the Lymphoma Study Group (1984–87). Br J Haematol. 1991;79(3):428–37.
12. Takatsuki K. Adult T-cell leukemia. New York: Oxford University Press; 1994.
13. Takatsuki K, Yamaguchi K, Kawano F, Hattori T, Nishimura H, Tsuda H, Sanada I, Nakada K, Itai Y. Clinical diversity in adult T-cell leukemia-lymphoma. Cancer Res. 1985;45:4644s–5s.

14. Tsukasaki K, Hermine O, Bazarbachi A, Ratner L, Ramos JC, Harrington Jr W, et al. Definition, prognostic factors, treatment, and response criteria of adult T-cell leukemia-lymphoma: a proposal from an international consensus meeting. J Clin Oncol. 2009;27:453–9.
15. Uchiyama T, Yodoi J, Sagawa K, Takatsuki K, Uchino H. Adult T-cell leukemia: clinical and hematologic features of 16 cases. Blood. 1977;50(3):481–92.
16. Volkman DJ, Popovic M, Gallo RC, Fauci AS. Human T cell leukemia/lymphoma virus-infected antigen-specific T cell clones: indiscriminant helper function and lymphokine production. J Immunol. 1985;34(6):4237–43.
17. Yamada Y, Kamihira S, Murata K, Yamamura M, Maeda T, Tsukasaki K, Jubash T, Atogami S, Sohda H, Taguchi T, Tomonaga M. Frequent hepatic involvement in adult T cell leukemia: comparison with non-Hodgkin's lymphoma. Leuk Lymphoma. 1997;26 (3–4):327–35.
18. Yamada Y, Atogami S, Hasegawa H, Kamihira S, Soda M, Satake M, et al. Nationwide survey of adult T-cell leukemia/lymphoma (ATL) in Japan. Rinsho Ketsueki. 2011;52:1765–71.
19. Yoshie O, Fujisawa R, Nakayama T, Harasawa H, Tago H, Izawa D, Hieshima K, Tatsumi Y, Matsushima K, Hasegawa H, Kanamaru A, Kamihira S, Yamada Y. Frequent expression of CCR4 in adult T-cell leukemia and human T-cell leukemia virus type 1-transformed T cells. Blood. 2002;99(5):1505–11.
20. Yoshida M, Miyoshi I, Hinuma Y. Isolation and characterization of retrovirus from cell lines of human adult T-cell leukemia and its implication in the disease. Proc Natl Acad Sci USA. 1982;79(6):2031–5.
21. Yoshida M, Seiki M, Yamaguchi K, Takatsuki K. Monoclonal integration of human T-cell leukemia provirus in all primary tumors of adult T-cell leukemia suggests causative role of human T-cell leukemia virus in the disease. Proc Natl Acad Sci USA. 1984;81(8):2534–7.

# Chapter 8
# Prognosis and Prognostic Index

Takuya Fukushima

## 8.1 Introduction

The classification of adult T-cell leukemia-lymphoma (ATL) into the acute, lymphoma, chronic, and smoldering types was proposed by Shimoyama and members of the Lymphoma Study Group based on prognostic factors, clinical features, and the natural history of the disease [1]. In that study, 818 ATL patients who were newly diagnosed between 1983 and 1987 were analyzed using this classification system. The median survival time (MST) was reported to be 6.2 months, 10.2 months, and 24.3 months for the acute, lymphoma, and chronic types, respectively, whereas the MST for the smoldering type had not yet been determined. The projected 2- and 4-year survival rates were 16.7% and 5.0% for the acute type, 21.3% and 5.7% for the lymphoma type, 52.4% and 26.9% for the chronic type, and 77.7% and 62.8% for the smoldering type, respectively (Fig. 8.1). Chronic-type ATL can be further categorized into the favorable and unfavorable subtypes according to the presence of either lactate dehydrogenase (LDH) or blood urea nitrogen (BUN) levels above the normal upper limit or an albumin level below the normal lower limit [2]. The acute, lymphoma, and unfavorable chronic types are defined as aggressive ATL, while the favorable chronic and smoldering types are defined as indolent ATL. These two categories of ATL are widely used to plan suitable therapeutic strategies.

T. Fukushima (✉)
Department of Clinical Laboratory Sciences, School of Health Sciences, University of the Ryukyus, Okinawa, Japan
e-mail: fukutaku@med.u-ryukyu.ac.jp



T. Watanabe, T. Fukushima (eds.), *Adult T-cell Leukemia/Lymphoma*,
DOI 10.1007/978-4-431-56523-9_8

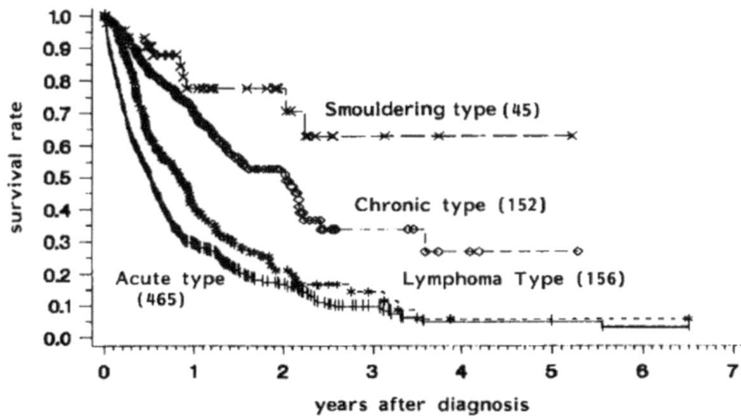


**Fig. 8.1** Survival curves of patients with adult T-cell leukemia-lymphoma (ATL) according to clinical subtype [1]

## 8.2 Prognosis of Aggressive ATL

The MST of patients with aggressive ATL in the 1980s has been reported to be approximately 8 months, with a 2-year survival rate of <5%. This was because this category of aggressive ATL is associated with a multidrug-resistant phenotype of malignant tumor cells, rapid proliferation of the tumor cells, a large tumor burden with multi-organ failure, hypercalcemia, and/or occurrence of frequent opportunistic infections [1–4]. The Japan Clinical Oncology Group (JCOG)-Lymphoma Study Group has conducted consecutive clinical trials to improve the survival of patients with aggressive ATL. Earlier trials (JCOG7801, JCOG8101, and JCOG8701) showed that the prognosis of aggressive ATL is worse than that of other types of non-Hodgkin lymphomas (Fig. 8.2) [5, 6]. After the classification system for ATL was established, three JCOG trials were conducted to test new therapeutic agents exclusively targeting aggressive ATL. The first phase II trial, JCOG9101 (1991–1993), evaluated combination chemotherapy with deoxycoformycin, an inhibitor of adenosine deaminase, which has been shown to be effective as monotherapy against relapsed and refractory ATL. However, the results were disappointing, with an MST of 7 months [7]. The next phase II trial, JCOG9303 (1994–1996), evaluated the chemotherapy regimen VCAP–AMP–VECP against aggressive ATL, with VCAP comprising vincristine (VCR), cyclophosphamide (CPA), doxorubicin (DXR), and prednisone (PSL); AMP comprising DXR, ranimustine, and PSL; and VECP comprising vindesine, etoposide, carboplatin, and PSL. This phase II trial showed promising results, with an MST of 13 months at the expense of hematological and other toxicities (Fig. 8.3.) [8]. In the light of these findings, the phase III trial, JCOG9801 (1998–2003), was conducted to compare a modified VCAP–AMP–VECP regimen versus the CHOP (CPA, VCR, DXR, and PSL)-14 regimen. The 3-year overall survival (OS) was higher in the modified

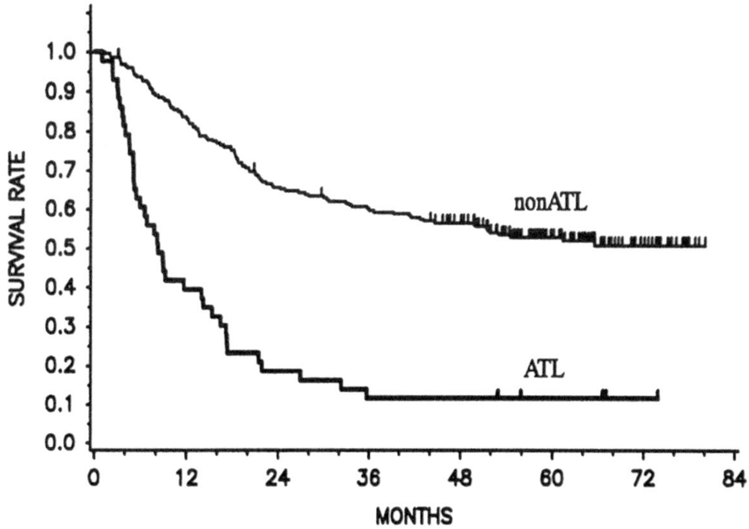


**Fig. 8.2** Comparison of the survival curves of ATL and non-ATL in JCOG8701 [6]

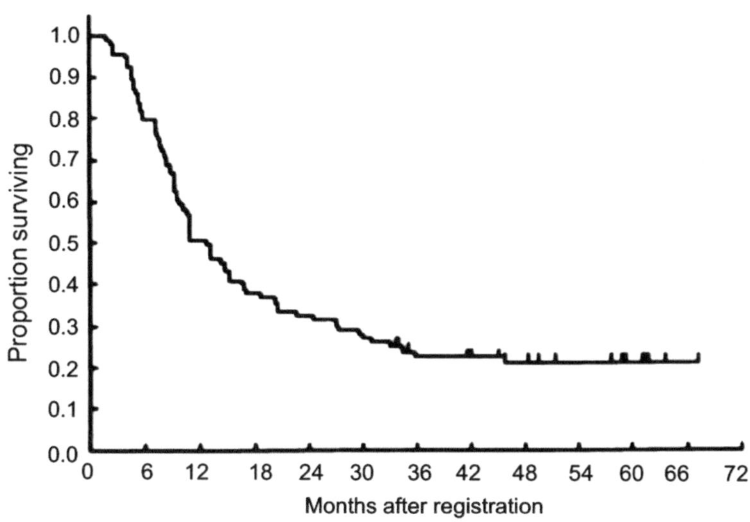


**Fig. 8.3** Kaplan–Meier estimate of the overall survival for the 93 eligible patients in JCOG9303 [8]

VCAP-AMP-VECP arm than in the CHOP-14 arm (24% vs. 13%), suggesting that the former is the more effective regimen at the expense of high toxicity for patients with newly diagnosed aggressive ATL (Fig. 8.4) [9].

The results of these three JCOG trials among patients with aggressive ATL led to an improvement in the 5-year OS among such patients from 5% in the 1980s to 15%

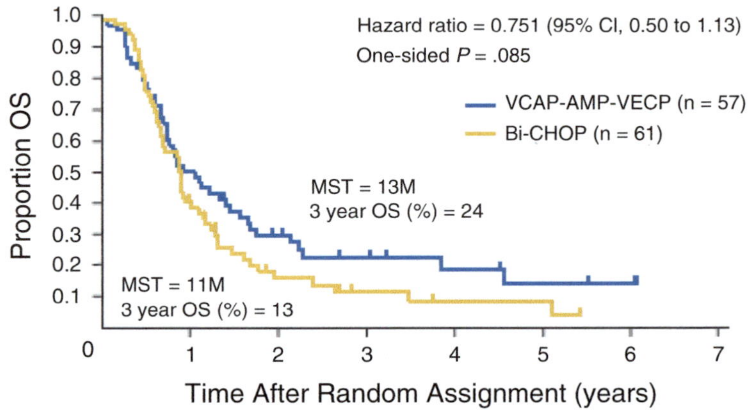


**Fig. 8.4** Kaplan–Meier estimate of overall survival for all randomly assigned patients in JCOG9801 [9]

in the 1990s. However, the best MST after chemotherapy for such patients remains short at around 1 year.

## 8.3 Prognosis of Indolent ATL

A retrospective analysis conducted across 40 institutions in Kyushu and Okinawa, Japan, among 337 patients with the smoldering and chronic types of ATL revealed an MST of 5.7 and 3.6 years, respectively [1]. Subgroup analysis revealed that for the smoldering type of ATL, there was no difference in the MST between patients treated with chemotherapy and those managed with watchful waiting. In contrast, for the chronic type of ATL, the MST of the patients managed with watchful waiting was significantly greater than that of those treated with chemotherapy (7.4 years vs. 2.0 years). Considering these data, watchful waiting is recommended as the standard treatment for indolent ATL.

A retrospective analysis of 90 patients with newly diagnosed smoldering (25 patients) and chronic (65 patients) ATL who were treated between 1974 and 2003 at Nagasaki University Hospital revealed an MST of 4.1 years. Twelve patients survived for more than 10 years, 44 patients progressed to the acute type, and 63 patients died. The estimated 5-, 10-, and 15-year survival rates were 47.2%, 25.4%, and 14.1%, respectively, with the absence of any plateau in the survival curve (Fig. 8.5) [10]. In a multicenter follow-up study between 1988 and 1997 in Kyushu, the MST of 26 patients diagnosed with smoldering ATL was 7.3 years [11].

These data indicate that the prognosis of indolent ATL is poorer than expected, although some patients could survive for more than 10 years.

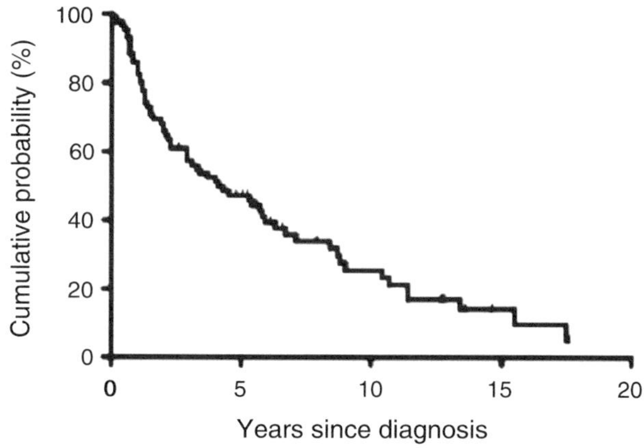


**Fig. 8.5** Overall survival of patients with indolent ATL [10]

## 8.4 Prognostic Index of Aggressive ATL

Several reports have been published on the risk factors for ATL. In a prospective randomized trial on advanced non-Hodgkin lymphoma conducted between 1981 and 1983, Shimoyama et al. found that poor performance status (PS) and high LDH levels are poor prognostic factors in patients with advanced T-cell leukemia-lymphoma, including ATL [5]. In a nationwide Japanese survey of 854 patients, multivariate analysis revealed that the major prognostic indicators of ATL are poor PS, high LDH levels, age ≥40 years, involvement of >3 lesions, and hypercalcemia [3]. These factors were then used to construct a risk model. Multivariate analysis identified the following additional factors associated with poor prognosis: thrombocytopenia [12], eosinophilia [13], bone marrow involvement [14], high interleukin (IL)-5 and IL-10 serum levels [15], C-C chemokine receptor 4 (CCR4) expression [16], lung resistance-related protein [17], TP-53 mutation [18], and CDKN2A deletion [12].

Recently, two types of prognostic indices (PIs) for aggressive ATL were published. A PI was defined for acute- and lymphoma-type ATL (ATL-PI) based on the findings of a retrospective analysis conducted in Japan between 2000 and 2009 using the medical records of 807 patients who did not receive allogeneic hematopoietic stem cell transplantation [19]. Multivariate analysis revealed the following independent and significant prognostic factors: Ann Arbor stage (I/II vs. III/IV), PS (0/1 vs. 2/3/4), age, serum albumin level, and soluble IL-2 receptor (IL-2R) expression. A simplified ATL-PI was established as follows:

| | | |
|---|---|---|
| Simplified ATL-PI | = | 2 (if stage = III/IV) |
| | | +1 (if ECOG PS >1) |
| | | +1 (if age >70 years) |
| | | +1 (if albumin <3.5 g/dL) |
| | | +1 (if sIL2-R>20,000 U/mL) |

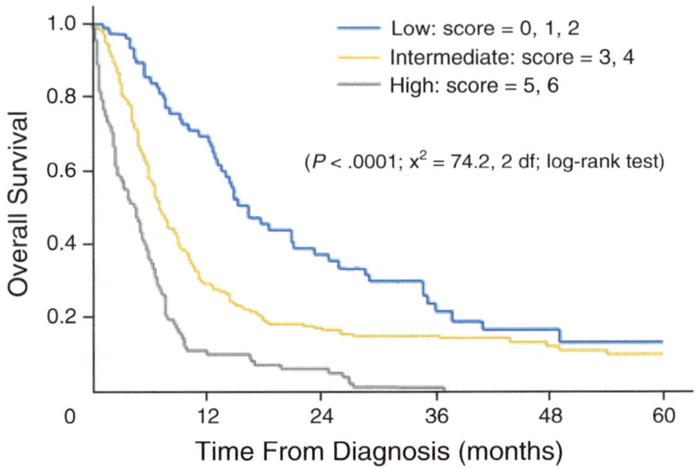


| No. at risk | | | | | | |
|---|---|---|---|---|---|---|
| Low | 77 | 45 | 22 | 11 | 6 | 3 |
| Intermediate | 208 | 52 | 26 | 18 | 14 | 9 |
| High | 118 | 10 | 6 | 2 | 0 | 0 |

**Fig. 8.6** Overall survival curves for the validation sample ($n = 403$) according to ATL-PI [19]

Patients with scores of 0–2 were categorized into the low-risk group, those with 3 and 4 into the intermediate-risk group, and those with 5 and 6 into the high-risk group. In the validation sample, the number of patients in the low-, intermediate-, and high-risk groups were 77 (19%), 208 (52%), and 118 (29%), respectively. The MST and 2-year OS were 16.2 months and 37%, 7.0 months and 17%, and 4.6 months and 6% in the low-, intermediate-, and high-risk groups, respectively (Fig. 8.6).

On the other hand, JCOG prospectively analyzed 276 patients with aggressive ATL (acute, lymphoma, and unfavorable chronic types) recruited from three prospective clinical trials (JCOG9109, JCOG9303, and JCOG9801) conducted after the introduction of the classification system for the clinical subtypes of ATL. Based on the results, the JCOG-PI was defined according to the corrected calcium levels and PS in the multivariate analysis of 193 patients [20]. On application of the JCOG-PI, the MST and 5-year OS were found to be 14 months and 18% in patients with both corrected calcium of <5.5 mEq/L and a PS of 0 or 1 (moderate risk) and 8 months and 4% in patients with corrected calcium of ≥5.5 mEq/L and/or a PS of 2–4 (high-risk group), respectively (Fig. 8.7). External validation of 127 evaluable patients revealed that the MST was 18 months and 6 months in the moderate- and high-risk groups, respectively, and the JCOG-PI showed good reproducibility.

Thus, both types of PIs for aggressive ATL are valuable tools for identifying patients with extremely poor prognosis and will be useful for the design of future studies on the combinations of new drugs or investigational strategies. However, the 5-year OS rates noted in both the studies were less than 15%, even in the group

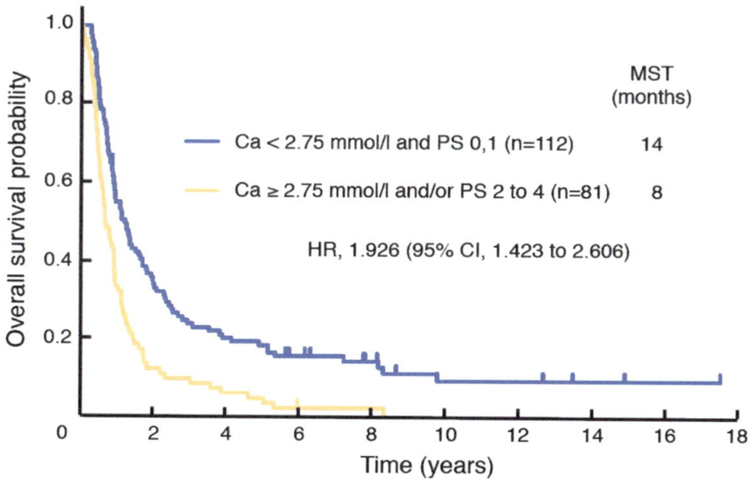


**Fig. 8.7** Overall survival curve of the patients in the training set according to JCOG-PI [20]

with better prognosis; therefore, the subgroup of patients with relatively favorable prognosis could not be identified using these tools. Future studies accounting for the use of molecular markers are necessary to identity factors indicating a favorable prognosis in patients with aggressive ATL.

## References


1. Shimoyama M. Diagnostic criteria and classification of clinical subtypes of adult T-cell leukaemia-lymphoma: a report from the Lymphoma Study Group (1984–1987). Br J Haematol. 1991;79:428–37.
2. Shimoyama M. Chemotherapy of ATL. In: Takatsuki K, editor. Adult T-cell leukemia. Oxford: Oxford University Press; 1994. p. 221–37.
3. Lymphoma Study Group. Major prognostic factors of patients with adult T-cell leukemia-lymphoma: a cooperative study-Lymphoma Study Group (1984–1987). Leuk Res. 1991;15:81–90.
4. Tobinai K, Watanabe T. Adult T-cell leukemia-lymphoma. In: Abeloff MD, Armitage JO, Niederhuber JE, Kastan MCB, editors. Clinical oncology. 3rd ed. Philadelphia: Elsevier Churchill Livingstone. p. 3109–30.
5. Shimoyama M, Ota K, Kikuchi M, Yunoki K, Konda S, Takatsuki K, Ichimaru M, Ogawa M, Kimura I, Tominaga S. Chemotherapeutic results and prognostic factors of patients with advanced non-Hodgkin's lymphoma treated with VEPA or VEPA-M. J Clin Oncol. 1988;6:128–41.
6. Tobibai K, Shimoyama M, Minato K, Shirakawa S, Kobayashi T, Hotta T. Japan Clinical Oncology Group phase II trial of second-generation "LSG4 protocol" in aggressive T- and B-lymphoma: a new predictive model for T- and B-lymphoma. Proc Am Soc Clin Oncol. 1994;13:378.
7. Tsukasaki K, Tobinai K, Shimoyama M, Kozuru M, Uike N, Yamada Y, Tomonaga M, Araki K, Kasai M, Takatsuki K, Tara M, Mikuni C, Hotta T, Lymphoma Study Group of the Japan Clinical Oncology Group. Deoxycoformycin-containing combination chemotherapy for

adult T-cell leukemia-lymphoma: Japan Clinical Oncology Group Study (JCOG9109). Int J Hematol. 2003;77:164–70.
8. Yamada Y, Tomonaga M, Fukuda H, Hanada S, Utsunomiya A, Tara M, Sano M, Ikeda S, Takatsuki K, Kozuru M, Araki K, Kawano F, Niimi M, Tobinai K, Hotta T, Shimoyama M. A new G-CSF supported combination chemotherapy, LSG15, for adult T-cell leukaemia-lymphoma: Japan Clinical Oncology Group Study 9303. Br J Haematol. 2001;113:375–82.
9. Tsukasaki K, Utsunomiya A, Fukuda H, Shibata T, Fukushima T, Takatsuka Y, Ikeda S, Masuda M, Nagoshi H, Ueda R, Tamura K, Sano M, Momita S, Yamaguchi K, Kawano F, Hanada S, Tobinai K, Shimoyama M, Hotta T, Tomonaga M, Japan Clinical Oncology Group Study JCOG9801. VCAP-AMP-VECP compared with biweekly CHOP for adult T-cell leukemia-lymphoma: Japan Clinical Oncology Group Study JCOG9801. J Clin Oncol. 2007;25:5458–64.
10. Takasaki Y, Iwanaga M, Imaizumi Y, Tawara M, Joh T, Kohno T, Yamada Y, Kamihira S, Ikeda S, Miyazaki Y, Tomonaga M, Tsukasaki K. Long-term study of indolent adult T-cell leukemia-lymphoma. Blood. 2010;115:4337–43.
11. Ishitsuka K, Ikeda S, Utsunomiya A, Saburi Y, Uozumi K, Tsukasaki K, Etou K, Muta K, Kinosita K, Tamura K. Smouldering adult T-cell leukaemia/lymphoma: a follow-up study in Kyushu. Br J Haematol. 2008;143:442–4.
12. Yamada Y, Hatta Y, Murata K, Sugawara K, Ikeda S, Mine M, Maeda T, Hirakata Y, Kamihira S, Tsukasaki K, Ogawa S, Hirai H, Koeffler HP, Tomonaga M. Deletion of p15 and/or p16 genes as a poor-prognosis factor in adult T-cell leukemia. J Clin Oncol. 1997;15:1778–85.
13. Utsunomiya A, Ishida T, Inagaki A, Yano H, Komatsu H, Iida S, Yonekura K, Takeuchi S, Takatsuka Y, Ueda R. Clinical significance of a blood eosinophilia in adult T-cell leukemia/lymphoma: a blood eosinophilia is a significant unfavorable prognostic factor. Leuk Res. 2007;31:915–20.
14. Takasaki Y, Iwanaga M, Tsukasaki K, Kusano M, Sugahara K, Yamada Y, Kamihira S, Ikeda S, Tomonaga M. Impact of visceral involvement and blood cell count abnormalities on survival in adult T-cell leukemia/lymphoma (ATLL). Leuk Res. 2007;31:751–7.
15. Inagaki A, Ishida T, Ishii T, Komatsu H, Iida S, Ding J, Yonekura K, Takeuchi S, Takatsuka Y, Utsunomiya A, Ueda R. Clinical significance of serum Th1-, Th2- and regulatory T cells-associated cytokines in adult T-cell leukemia/lymphoma: high interleukin-5 and -10 levels are significant unfavorable prognostic factors. Int J Cancer. 2006;118:3054–61.
16. Ishida T, Utsunomiya A, Iida S, Inagaki H, Takatsuka Y, Kusumoto S, Takeuchi G, Shimizu S, Ito M, Komatsu H, Wakita A, Eimoto T, Matsushita K, Ueda R. Clinical significance of CCR4 expression in adult T-cell leukemia/lymphoma: its close association with skin involvement and unfavorable outcome. Clin Cancer Res. 2003;9:3625–34.
17. Ohno N, Tani A, Uozumi K, Hanada S, Furukawa T, Akiba S, Sumizawa T, Utsunomiya A, Arima T, Akiyama S. Expression of functional lung resistance-related protein predicts poor outcome in adult T-cell leukemia. Blood. 2001;98:1160–5.
18. Tawara M, Hogerzeil SJ, Yamada Y, Yakasaki Y, Soda H, Hasegawa H, Murata K, Ikeda S, Imaizumi Y, Sugahara K, Tsuruda K, Tsukasaki K, Tomonaga M, Hirakata Y, Kamihira S. Impact of p53 aberration on the progression of adult T-cell leukemia/lymphoma. Cancer Lett. 2006;234:249–55.
19. Katsuya H, Yamanaka T, Ishitsuka K, Utsunomiya A, Sasaki H, Hanada S, Eto T, Moriuchi Y, Saburi Y, Miyahara M, Sueoka E, Uike N, Yoshida S, Yamashita K, Tsukasaki K, Suzushima H, Ohno Y, Matsuoka H, Jo T, Suzumiya J, Tamura K. Prognostic index for acute- and lymphoma-type adult T-cell leukemia/lymphoma. J Clin Oncol. 2012;30:1635–40.
20. Fukushima T, Nomura S, Shimoyama M, Shibata T, Imaizumi Y, Moriuchi Y, Tomoyose T, Uozumi K, Kobayashi Y, Fukushima N, Utsunomiya A, Tara M, Nosaka K, Hidaka M, Uike N, Yoshida S, Tamura K, Ishitsuka K, Kurosawa M, Nakata M, Fukuda H, Hotta T, Tobinai K, Tsukasaki K. Japan Clinical Oncology Group (JCOG) prognostic index and characterization of long-term survivors of aggressive adult T-cell leukaemia-lymphoma (JCOG0902A). Br J Haematol. 2014;166:739–48.

# Chapter 9
# Treatment of Indolent Adult T-cell Leukemia/Lymphoma (ATL)

**Kenji Ishitsuka**

## 9.1 Treatment of Indolent Adult T-cell Leukemia/Lymphoma (ATL)

### *9.1.1 Definition of Indolent ATL*

Based on prognostic factors, clinical features, and natural history of the disease, ATL is divided into four clinical subtypes: acute type, lymphoma type, chronic type, and smoldering type [16]. Chronic ATL can be further divided into "favorable" and "unfavorable" subtypes based on either LDH or BUN levels above the normal upper limits or albumin level below the normal lower limit [17]. The acute, lymphoma, and unfavorable chronic types are classified as aggressive ATL and have median survival times (MSTs) of 6, 10, and 15 months, respectively. However, the smoldering and favorable chronic types, which have 4-year survival rates (OS) of 70% and 63%, respectively, are instead classified as indolent ATL.

### *9.1.2 Clinical Course of Indolent ATL*

Several large-cohort retrospective analyses for patients with indolent ATL have been reported from Japan. Retrospective analysis of 337 patients with chronic and smoldering ATL at 40 institutions based in Kyushu and Okinawa, Japan, demonstrated that the MSTs for each type were 3.6 years and 5.2 years, respectively [22]. Subgroup analysis revealed that there is no difference in survival time

K. Ishitsuka (✉)
Division of Hematology and Immunology, Center for Chronic Viral Disease, Graduate School of Medical and Dental Sciences, Kagoshima University, Kagoshima, Japan
e-mail: kenji-i@m.kufm.kagoshima-u.ac.jp



T. Watanabe, T. Fukushima (eds.), *Adult T-cell Leukemia/Lymphoma*,
DOI 10.1007/978-4-431-56523-9_9

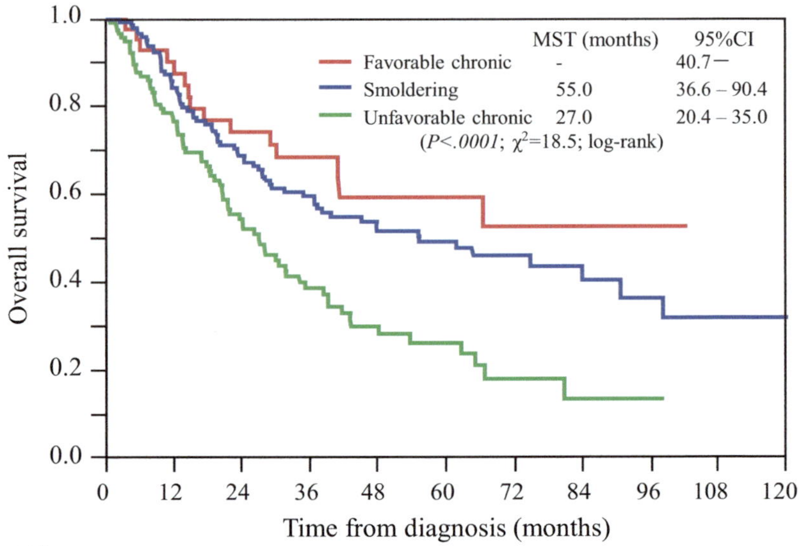


| No. at risk | | | | | | | | | | | |
|---|---|---|---|---|---|---|---|---|---|---|---|
| Favorable chronic | 49 | 34 | 28 | 17 | 14 | 11 | 8 | 6 | 1 | 0 | 0 |
| Smoldering | 157 | 114 | 87 | 66 | 49 | 37 | 21 | 13 | 9 | 6 | 6 |
| Unfavorable chronic | 128 | 79 | 48 | 29 | 18 | 13 | 7 | 4 | 1 | 0 | 0 |

**Fig. 9.1** Overall survival in patients with chronic and smoldering ATL (From Katsuya et al. [12])

between watchful waiting and chemotherapy in patients with smoldering ATL, and that furthermore MST of the watchful waiting group was superior to that of the chemotherapy group in patients with chronic type (7.4 years vs 2.0 years).

Based on these data, watchful waiting is regarded as the standard treatment for patients with indolent ATL in Japan, as no benefits to early intervention with antineoplastic agents have been established. Meanwhile, in Europe and America, antiviral therapy with interferon-α and a retroviral agent, zidovudine (IFN/AZT), which is not covered under health insurance for ATL in Japan, is administered to patients with both indolent and acute ATL as standard treatment.

According to a recent Japanese nationwide survey, MST in patients with the smoldering type is 55 months with a 52% 4-year OS ($n = 157$). MST has not yet been elucidated for the favorable chronic type, but 4-year OS has been found to be 60% (Fig. 9.1) [12]. In this study, the MST of patients with smoldering ATL treated by hematologists was 36.7 months and that of those treated by dermatologists was 74.5 months. Most patients included in the study were followed by supportive care only—namely, watchful waiting—until progression to aggressive ATL. In another Japanese study from Nagasaki University, the MST for patients with smoldering ATL treated by hematologists was reported to be 34.8 months ($n = 25$) [19].

### *9.1.3 Treatment Strategy for Indolent ATL in an International Consensus Meeting*

An International Consensus Meeting has recommended treating patients with IFN/AZT or watchful waiting if patients are symptomatic or with watchful waiting alone if patients are asymptomatic [21].

#### 9.1.3.1 Watchful Waiting

As mentioned earlier, no study has reported benefits of early therapeutic intervention for patients with indolent ATL. A retrospective Japanese study failed to show the benefit of chemotherapy for patients with chronic ATL; in this study, MST was 2.0 years with chemotherapy ($n = 49$) and 7.4 years with watchful waiting ($n = 90$) [22]. Although there may be possible bias in determining the therapeutic modality due to the retrospective nature of the patient cohort, watchful waiting has been held to be the standard of care for this group of patients. This might be partly because clinicians were familiar with using a similar strategy for patients with early stage chronic lymphocytic leukemia.

The long-term study of 90 patients with indolent ATL in Nagasaki revealed that MST was 4.1 years; 12 patients remained alive for over 10 years, 44 progressed to acute ATL, and 60 patients died. The estimated 5-, 10-, and 15-year OSs were 47.2%, 25.4%, and 14.1%, respectively, with no plateau in survival curve [19]. In addition, the aforementioned Japanese retrospective study in 2015 showed that median time to introduction to systemic chemotherapy for smoldering and favorable chronic ATL were 56.0 months and 39.1 months, respectively (Fig. 9.2) [12].

Prognosis of indolent ATL with watchful waiting was poorer than expected, as about half of patients progressed to aggressive ATL. Further studies of indolent ATL are required to develop effective treatments for preventing progression to aggressive ATL.

#### 9.1.3.2 Local Therapy

Some patients with indolent ATL have skin lesions. These can be treated with skin-directed therapy for relief of symptoms as well as cosmetic purposes, such as topical steroids, narrow-band ultraviolet B, psoralen photochemotherapy, electron beam therapy, and radiation therapy. A retrospective analysis of ten consecutive ATL patients at the National Institutes of Health between 1997 and 2010, including two patients with smoldering ATL treated with radiotherapy, demonstrated that all 20 lesions (cutaneous = 10, nodal = 8, extranodal = 2) responded to therapy, with in-field complete responses in 40% of lesions [20]. Although no report has yet revealed clear evidence about the effectiveness of local therapy for skin lesions, radiotherapy could be considered in symptomatic local progression of ATL.

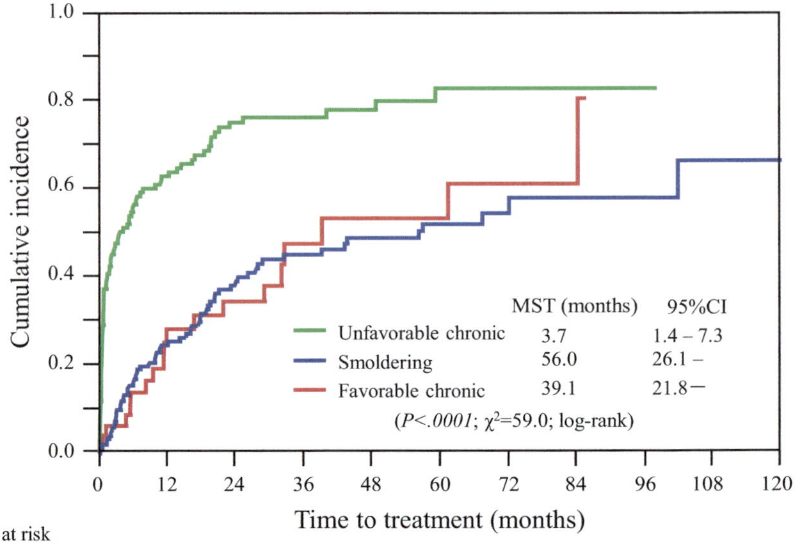


| No. at risk | | | | | | | | | | | |
|---|---|---|---|---|---|---|---|---|---|---|---|
| Unfavorable chronic | 128 | 41 | 23 | 18 | 12 | 7 | 4 | 1 | 0 | 0 | 0 |
| Smoldering | 157 | 90 | 66 | 52 | 37 | 27 | 13 | 10 | 7 | 4 | 4 |
| Favorable chronic | 49 | 25 | 21 | 10 | 9 | 7 | 4 | 3 | 0 | 0 | 0 |

**Fig. 9.2** Cumulative incidence of the introduction of systemic chemotherapy in patients with chronic and smoldering ATL (From Katsuya et al. [12])

However, the benefits of these approaches on the eventual prognosis are unknown [12, 18].

#### 9.1.3.3 Chemotherapy

Currently, there exist no curative treatment procedures for ATL except for allogeneic hematopoietic stem cell transplantation. In addition, early introduction of chemotherapy for patients with indolent ATL is not currently supported by any solid data regarding any potential positive or negative effects on survival. Early introduction of chemotherapy might prolong progression-free survival but not necessarily overall survival, and it is at the expense of toxicities that are similar to the experiences of patients with low-grade lymphoma [22].

Systemic therapy such as steroids, oral retinoids, interferon-γ, or single-agent chemotherapy, for example, with oral etoposide, may be applied for relief of symptoms as well as cosmetic purposes; however, the beneficial effects of these approaches on the eventual prognosis of the patients are also not yet confirmed [18].

#### 9.1.3.4 Interferon-α and Antiretroviral Agents

In several small series of patients, interferon-α monotherapy produced complete remission in less than 10%, although occasional durable responses have been reported [6, 9, 11, 14]. Shibata et al. found that the combination of interferon-α and an antiretroviral agent such as zidovudine (IFN/AZT) induced a rapid and durable response in a patient with ATL who was coinfected with both HIV type I and human T-cell leukemia virus type I (HTLV-1) [23]. Based on these data, two preliminary phase II studies were conducted, and a high response rate was observed in previously untreated acute ATL [3, 4]. The efficacy of IFN/AZT was confirmed in a French trial that included 19 newly diagnosed patients with ATL and in a UK clinical trial that included 15 patients with ATL [5, 15]. A retrospective meta-analysis reported 5-year OS of 100% and 42% in patients with chronic and smoldering ATL treated by IFN/AZT and chemotherapy, respectively (Fig. 9.3) [1]. The number of patients included in this analysis was very small, and possible bias, such as heterogeneity of the decision process for selecting the therapeutic modality for each patient and unreliable information of maintenance therapy and second-line chemotherapy [7] due to its retrospective nature, cannot be avoided. However, the results of IFN/AZT in patients with smoldering and chronic ATL were promising in light of potentially establishing a new effective ATL treatment. Considering the promising but preliminary nature of the findings by Bazarbachi et al. [1], the Japan Clinical Oncology Group-Lymphoma Study Group (JCOG-LSG) has started a phase III study comparing IFN/AZT with watchful waiting for

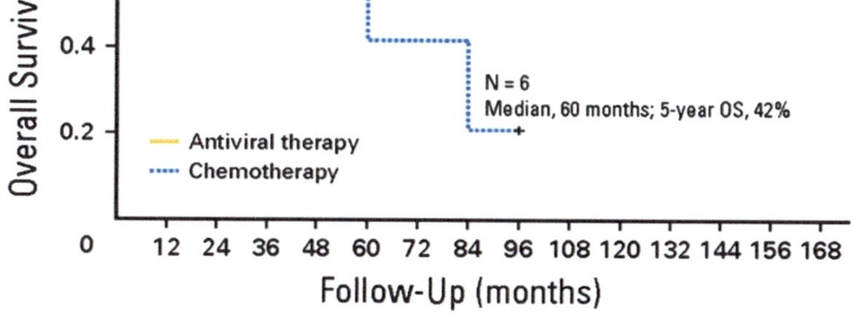


Fig. 9.3 Overall survival in patients with chronic and smoldering ATL treated with either chemotherapy or antiretroviral therapy represented by combination of interferon-α and zidovudine, observed in a retrospective study [1]

indolent ATL (JCOG1111; UMIN000011805). This study may validate the efficacy of early intervention for indolent ATL by IFN/AZT in Japanese populations.

Several suggested mechanisms of the anti-ATL effects induced by IFN/AZT have been reported; however, these effects must be clarified further [8]. The feasibility and efficacy of combination of arsenic trioxide and IFN/AZT have also been reported in a small number of patients with chronic ATL [13]; however, these results are also in need of confirmation by larger prospective studies.

### *9.1.4 Further Perspectives*

The standard of care for indolent ATL in Japan has been watchful waiting, while recent international studies have suggested the potential for prolonging survival with combination therapy with interferon-α and antiretroviral drugs. Moreover, two recent Japanese retrospective studies [12, 19] indicated that indolent ATL, especially smoldering ATL, has poorer prognosis than that reported in former studies [16]. Taken together, efforts toward innovative treatment are warranted to improve the prognosis for indolent ATL without sacrificing patients' quality of life. Two approaches can be considered for possible improvement of the outcome for patients with indolent ATL. One is to stratify patients who should have early intervention by elucidating prognostic factors in indolent ATL. The second is to develop an optimal treatment based on the risk-stratified approach. Combination of interferon-α and antiretroviral therapy is one option, with other possible modalities such as immunological approach by vaccination, use of mogamulizumab (a defucosylated humanized C-C chemokine receptor 4 antibody), and use of immunomodulatory drugs, as well as novel chemotherapeutics such as pralatrexate (a folate analogue metabolic inhibitor) and forodesine (a transition-state analogue of purine nucleoside phosphorylase), which have been introduced or are in clinical trials for aggressive ATL and/or peripheral T-cell lymphoma.

Recently, integrated molecular analysis for patients with ATL has revealed that somatic alterations affected highly enriched T-cell receptor/NF-κB signaling, G protein-coupled receptors associated with T-cell migration, and other T-cell-related pathways, as well as immune surveillance-related genes [10]. Another study on epigenetic landscape of ATL cells has revealed that ATL cells are characterized by Polycomb Repressive Complex 2 (PRC2) hyperactivation with genome-wide histone 3 lysine 27 trimethylation (H3K27 me3) accumulation [2]. A new agent that inhibits both histone methylases EZH1 and EZH2 that are the components of PRC2 can induce cell death of ATL cells as well as HTLV-1-infected cells [2]. Clinical study is now underway for this dual inhibitor of EZH1/2. Further studies are ongoing to detect genes associated with the progression from indolent to aggressive disease. The development of new agents for target genes specific to indolent ATL, which may become clear as a result of these studies, in addition to well-designed clinical studies involving international collaboration is needed to overcome this incurable, heterogeneous, and rare disease.

## References

1. Bazarbachi A, Plumelle Y, Ramos CJ, Tortevoye P, Otrock Z, Taylor C, Gessain A, Harrington W, Panelatti G, Hermine O. Meta-analysis on the use of Zidovudine and interferon-alfa in adult T-cell leukemia/lymphoma showing improved survival in the leukemic subtypes. J Clin Oncol. 2010;28(27):4177–83.
2. Fujikawa D, Nakagawa S, Hori M, Kurokawa N, Soejima A, Nakano K, Yamochi T, Nakashima M, Kobayashi S, Tanaka Y, Iwanaga M, Utsunomiya A, Uchimaru K, Yamagishi M, Watanabe T. Polycomb-dependent epigenetic landscape in adult T-cell leukemia. Blood. 2016;127(14):1790–802.
3. Gill PS, Harrington Jr W, Kaplan MH, Ribeiro RC, Bennett JM, Liebman HA, Bernstein-Singer M, Espina BM, Gabral L, Allen S, Kornblau S, Pike MC, Levine AM. Treatment of adult T-cell leukemia-lymphoma with a combination of interferon alfa and zidovudine. N Engl J Med. 1995;113:779–84.
4. Hermine O, Bouscary D, Gessain A, Turlure P, Leblond V, Franck N, Buzyn-Veil A, Rio B, Macintyre E, Dreyfus F, Bazarbachi A. Treatment of adult T-cell leukemia-lymphoma with zidovudine and interferon alfa. N Engl J Med. 1995;332:1749–51.
5. Hermine O, Allard I, Levy V, Arnulf B, Gessain A, Bazarbachi A. A prospective phase II clinical trial with the use of zidovudine and interferon-alpha in the cute and lymphoma forms of adult T-cell leukemia/lymphoma. Hematol J. 2002;3:276–82.
6. Ichimaru M, Kamihira S, Moriuchi Y, Kuraishi Y, Usui N, Toki H, Okabe Y, Shibuya T, Umei T. Clinical study on the effect of natural alpha-interferon (HLBI) in the treatment of adult T-cell leukemia. Jpn J Cancer Chemother. 1988;15:2975–81. (In Japanese)
7. Ishitsuka K, Fukushima T, Tsukasaki K, Tobinai K. Is Zidovudine and interferon-alfa the gold standard for adult T-cell leukemia-lymphoma? J Clin Oncol. 2010;28:e765.
8. Ishitsuka K, Tsukasaki K, Tamura K. Interferon alfa and antiretroviral agents: a treatment option for adult T-cell leukemia/lymphoma. Drugs Today (Barc). 2011;47(8):615–23.
9. Kamihira S, Soda H, Kinoshita K, Ichimaru M. Effect of human lymphoblast interferon in adult T-cell leukemia and non-Hodgkin's lymphoma. Jpn J Cancer Chemother. 1983;10:2188–93. (In Japanese)
10. Kataoka K, Nagata Y, Kitanaka A, Shiraishi Y, Shimamura T, Yasunaga J, Totoki Y, Chiba K, Sato-Otsubo A, Nagae G, Ishii R, Muto S, Kotani S, Watatani Y, Takeda J, Sanada M, Tanaka H, Suzuki H, Sato Y, Shiozawa Y, Yoshizato T, Yoshida K, Makishima H, Iwanaga M, Ma G, Nosaka K, Hishizawa M, Itonaga H, Imaizumi Y, Munakata W, Ogasawara H, Sato T, Sasai K, Muramoto K, Penova M, Kawaguchi T, Nakamura H, Hama N, Shide K, Kubuki Y, Hidaka T, Kameda T, Nakamaki T, Ishiyama K, Miyawaki S, Yoon SS, Tobinai K, Miyazaki Y, Takaori-Kondo A, Matsuda F, Takeuchi K, Nureki O, Aburatani H, Watanabe T, Shibata T, Matsuoka M, Miyano S, Shimoda K, Ogawa S. Integrated molecular analysis of adult T-cell leukemia/lymphoma. Nat Genet. 2015;47:1304–15.
11. Kimura K. Cooperative Study Group of Ro 22-8181 in Japan. Phase II study of recombinant leukocyte A interferon (Ro 22-8181) in hematological malignancies. Jpn J Cancer Chemother. 1985;12:928–35. (In Japanese)
12. Katsuya H, Ishitsuka K, Utsunomiya A, Hanada S, Eto T, Moriuchi Y, Saburi Y, Miyahara M, Sueoka E, Uike N, Yoshida S, Ymashita K, Tsukasaki K, Suzushima H, Ohno Y, Matsuoka H, Jo T, Amano M, Hino R, Shimokawa M, Kawai K, Suzumiya J, Tamura K. Treatment and survival among 1594 patients with ATL. Blood. 2015;126:2570–7.
13. Kochour G, Tarhini M, Kooshyar MM, El Hajj H, Wattel E, Mahmoudi M, Hatoum H, Rahimi H, Maleki M, Rafatpanah H, Rahim Rezaee SA, Yazdi MT, Shirdel A, de The H, Hermine O, Farid R, Bazarbachi A. Phase 2 study of the efficacy and safety of the combination of arsenic trioxide, interferon alpha, and zidovudine in newly diagnosed chronic adult T-cell leukemia/lymphoma (ATL). Blood. 2009;113:6528–32.

14. Matsumura M, Yoneyama A, Nakamura T, Higashihara M, Yotami Y, Tanabe A, Ohashi T, Oka H, Nakahara K. A first case of complete remission of β-interferon sensitive adult T-cell leukemia. Eur J Haematol. 1987;39:282–7.
15. Matutes E, Taylor GP, Gavenagh J, Pagliuca A, Bareford D, Domingo A, Hamblin M, Kelsey S, Mir N, Reilly JT. Interferon α and zidovudine therapy in adult T-cell leukaemia lymphoma: response and outcome in 15 patients. Br J Haematol. 2001;113:779–84.
16. Shimoyama M. Diagnostic criteria and classification of clinical subtypes of adult T-cell leukaemia-lymphoma. A report from the Lymphoma Study Group (1984–87). Br J Haematol. 1991;79:428–37.
17. Shimoyama M. Chemotherapy of ATL. In: Takatsuki K, editor. Adult T-cell leukemia. Oxford: Oxford University Press; 1994. p. 221–37.
18. Sugaya M, Hamada T, Kawai K, Yonekura K, Ohtsuka M, Shimauchi T, Tokura Y, Nozaki K, Isutsu K, Suzuki R, Setoyama M, Nagatani T, Koga H, Tani M, Iwatsuki K. Guideline for the management of cutaneous lymphoma (2011): a consensus statement by the Japanese Skin Cancer Society – Lymphoma Study Group. J Dermatol. 2013;40:2–14.
19. Takasaki Y, Iwanaga M, Imaizumi Y, Tawara M, Joh T, Kohno T, Yamada Y, Kamihira S, Ikeda S, Miyazaki Y, Tomonaga M, Tsukasaki K. Long-term study of indolent adult T-cell leukemia-lymphoma. Blood. 2010;115:4337–43.
20. Simone 2nd CBII, Morris JC, Stewart DM, Urquhart NE, Janik JE, Kreitman RJ, Lita E, Conlon K, Wharfe G, Waldmann TA, Kaushal A. Radiation therapy for the management of patients with HTLV-1-associated adult T-cell leukemia/lymphoma. Blood. 2012;120:1816–9.
21. Tsukasaki K, Hermine O, Bazarbachi A, Tatner L, Ramos JC, Harrington Jr W, O'Mahony D, Janik JE, Bitterncourt AL, Taylor GP, Yamaguchi K, Utsunomiya A, Tobinai K, Watanabe T. Definition, prognostic factors, treatment, and response criteria of adult T-cell leukemia-lymphoma: a proposal from an international consensus meeting. J Clin Oncol. 2009;27:453–9.
22. Yamada Y. High-risk aggressive lymphoma (ATL). Rinsho Ketsueki. 2001;42:293–8. (In Japanese)
23. Shibata D, Brynes RK, Rabinowitz A, Hanson CA, Slovak ML, Spira TJ, Gill P. Human T-cell lymphotropic virus type I (HTLV-I)-associated adult T-cell leukemia-lymphoma in a patient infected with human immunodeficiency virus type 1 (HIV-1). Ann Intern Med. 1989;111 (11):871–5.

# Chapter 10
# Chemotherapy of Aggressive Adult T-cell Leukemia/Lymphoma (ATL)

**Kunihiro Tsukasaki**

## 10.1 Development of Chemotherapy for Aggressive Adult T-cell Leukemia-Lymphoma (ATL)

The recent International T-Cell Lymphoma Project on 1314 patients revealed that ATL was the fourth most common T-cell lymphoma, mainly in Asia, especially Japan, and the prognosis was worst among the T-cell lymphomas [5]. The poor prognosis is associated with the multidrug resistance of ATL cells, high tumor burden with multi-organ involvement, complicated immunodeficiency and hypercalcemia, and advanced age at onset [1].

Since 1978, chemotherapy trials have been consecutively conducted for patients newly diagnosed with aggressive non-Hodgkin lymphoma including ATL by JCOG's Lymphoma Study Group (LSG), and the following results were obtained for this disease (Table 10.1) [4]. The first trial, called LSG1 (1978–1980), utilized VEPA therapy, which consisted of vincristine (VCR), cyclophosphamide (CPA), prednisolone (PSL), and doxorubicin (DOX) [6]. In this study, patients with NHL (including ATL) at an advanced stage were enrolled. The complete remission (CR) rate was lowest (18%) for ATL, intermediate (36%) for peripheral non-ATL T-cell lymphoma (PNTL), and highest (64%) for B-cell lymphoma [4]. Between 1981 and 1983, the JCOG-LSG conducted a phase III trial using LSG1-VEPA versus LSG2-VEPA-M (VEPA + methotrexate) against advanced NHL, including ATL [7]. Patients' sera were examined for anti-HTLV-1 antibody to distinguish ATL from PNTL. The CR rate for patients who were given LSG2-VEPA-M for ATL (37%) was higher than that for patients who were given LSG1-VEPA (17%; $P = 0.09$). In the LSG1/LSG2 trial, however, the CR rate was significantly lower for ATL than for B-cell lymphoma and PNTL ($P < 0.001$). The MST of the

K. Tsukasaki (✉)
Department of Hematology, National Cancer Center Hospital East, Kashiwa, Japan
e-mail: ktsukasa@east.ncc.go.jp



T. Watanabe, T. Fukushima (eds.), *Adult T-cell Leukemia/Lymphoma*,
DOI 10.1007/978-4-431-56523-9_10

**Table 10.1** Results of the JCOG-LSG trials for adult T-cell leukemia-lymphoma (ATL)

| Protocol | Regimen | Phase | No. of pts | %CR | MST (mo) | Survival (%) | Refs. |
|---|---|---|---|---|---|---|---|
| JCOG7801 | VEPA | II | 18 | 17 | 5 | 0 (3 years) | [6] |
| JCOG8101 | | III | 54 | 28 | 7.5 | 8.3 (4 years) | [7] |
| | VEPA | | 24 | 17 | NA | NA | |
| | VEPAM | | 30 | 37 | NA | NA | |
| JCOG8701 | LSG4 | II | 42 | 43 | 8 | 12 (5 years) | [9] |
| JCOG9109 | LSG11 | II | 60 | 28 | 7 | 15.5 (2 years) | [10] |
| JCOG9303 | LSG15 | II | 93 | 35 | 13 | 31 (2 years) | [11] |
| JCOG9801 | | III | 118 | | | | [2] |
| | mLSG15 | | 57 | 40 | 13 | 24 (3 years) | |
| | CHOP-14 | | 61 | 25 | 11 | 13 (3 years) | |

54 patients with ATL treated with LSG1/LSG2 was 6 months, and the estimated 4-year survival rate was only 8% [7]. These results suggest that CHOP-like chemotherapy of the first generation was not very effective against ATL.

In 1987, JCOG initiated a multicenter phase II study (JCOG8701) of a multiagent combination chemotherapy (LSG4) for advanced aggressive NHL (including ATL). LSG4 consisted of three regimens: (1) VEPA-B (VEPA plus bleomycin), (2) M-FEPA (methotrexate, vindesine, cyclophosphamide, prednisone, and doxorubicin), and (3) VEPP-B, (vincristine, etoposide, procarbazine, prednisone, and bleomycin) [4, 8]. The CR rate (72%) for the LSG4 protocol among patients with aggressive NHL including ATL was significantly higher than that for the LSG1/LSG2 trial (57%; $P < 0.05$). The CR rate for ATL was improved from 28% (LSG1/LSG2) to 43% (LSG4). On the other hand, the CR rate for LSG4 was significantly lower for ATL than for B lymphoma and PNTL ($P < 0.01$). The patients with ATL still showed a poor prognosis, with an MST of 8 months and a 4-year survival rate of 12%; however, the CR rate was increased to 12% (5 of 43) compared with 4% (2 of 54) in the LSG1/LSG2 trial. A multivariate analysis of the 267 patients with advanced aggressive NHL who were treated with LSG4 demonstrated that the clinical diagnosis of ATL was the most significant unfavorable prognostic factor (relative risk: 3.19; $P = 0.0001$) for aggressive NHL patients in Japan [4, 8].

The disappointing results with conventional chemotherapies have led to a search for new active agents. Multicenter phase I and II studies of 2′-deoxycoformycin (DCF; pentostatin), a purine analog having irreversible inhibition activity of adenosine deaminase), were conducted against ATL in Japan. The phase II study revealed a response rate of 32% (10 of 31) in cases of relapsed or refractory ATL (2CRs and 8PRs) [9]. These encouraging results and the proposal of subtype classification of ATL by JCOG-LSG through nationwide survey of ATL prompted the Japanese investigators to conduct a phase II trial (JCOG9109; LSG11) of DCF-incorporated regimen with VCR, DOX, ETP, and PSL as initial chemotherapy exclusively for aggressive ATL [10]. Sixty-two previously untreated patients with ATL (34 acute, 21 lymphoma, and 7 unfavorable chronic type) were enrolled.

Among the 60 eligible patients, there were 17 CRs (28%) and 14 partial responses (PRs) (overall response rate [ORR] = 52%). The MST was 7.4 months, and the estimated 2-year survival rate was 17%. The prognosis of patients with ATL remained poor, even though they were treated with a pentostatin-containing combination chemotherapy.

In 1994, JCOG-LSG initiated a new multiagent combination phase II study (JCOG9303; LSG15): a nine-drug regimen consisting of VCR, CPA, DOX, PSL, nimustine (MCNU), VDS, ETP, and carboplatin (CBDCA) with the intrathecal administration of MTX and PSL, for untreated patients with ATL [11]. In this study, the elevation of relative dose intensity was attempted with the prophylactic use of granulocyte colony-stimulating factor (G-CSF). In addition, non-cross-resistant agents such as MCNU and CBDCA were incorporated into the regimens. Ninety-six previously untreated patients with aggressive ATL were enrolled: 58 with acute type, 28 with lymphoma type, and 10 with unfavorable chronic type. Of the 93 eligible patients, 81% responded (75 of 93), 33 patients (35%) achieving CR and 42 (45%) achieving PR. Patients with lymphoma-type ATL showed a better CR rate (67%, 18 of 27) than patients with acute-type ATL (20%, 11 of 56) and patients with unfavorable chronic-type ATL (40%, 4 of 10). The OS rate of 93 eligible patients at 2 years was 31%. The MST was 13 months, and the median follow-up duration of the 20 surviving patients was 4.2 years. A trend toward better survival for patients with lymphoma-type ATL (MST, 20 months) compared with patients with acute-type ATL (MST, 11 months) was recognized (hazard ratio: 1.65). Grade 4 hematologic toxicities of neutropenia and thrombocytopenia were observed in 65% and 53% of the patients, respectively, but grade 4 non-hematologic toxicity was observed in only one patient. It was concluded that LSG15 was feasible with mild non-hematologic toxicity, and that it has improved the clinical outcome of patients with ATL (Fig. 10.1).

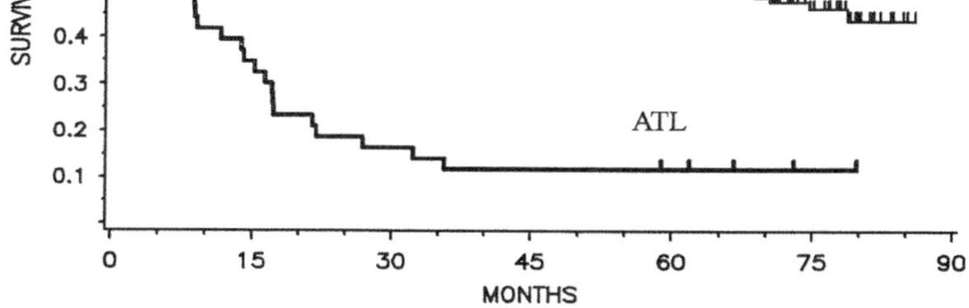


**Fig. 10.1** Kaplan-Meier estimate of overall survival (OS) for all patients with aggressive non-Hodgkin lymphoma treated with LSG4 in relation to disease entity. *ATL* adult T-cell leukemia-lymphoma

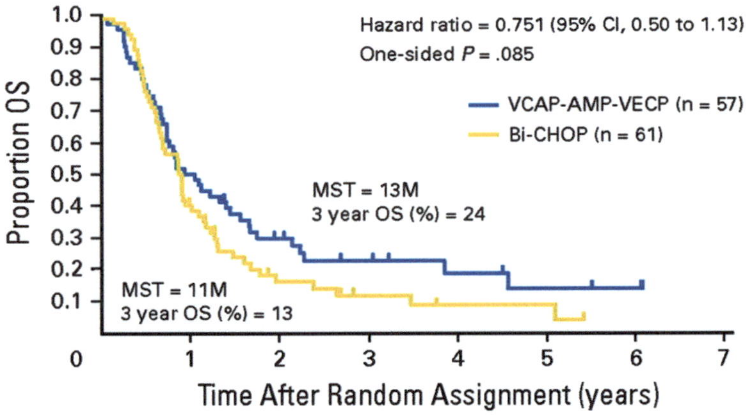


**Fig. 10.2** Kaplan-Meier estimate of overall survival (OS) for all randomly assigned patients in JCOG9801 study in relation to treatment regimen

To confirm whether LSG15 is a new standard for the treatment of aggressive ATL, JCOG-LSG conducted a phase III study comparing mLSG15 and CHOP-14 (CPA, DOX, VCR, and PSL) [2]. Previously untreated patients with aggressive ATL were randomly assigned to receive either six courses of LSG15 every 4 weeks or eight courses of CHOP-14. Both regimens were supported with G-CSF and intrathecal prophylaxis. mLSG15 in JCOG9801 was a modified version of LSG15 in JCOG9303, consisting of three regimens: VCAP [VCR 1 mg/m$^2$ (maximum 2 mg), CPA 350 mg/m$^2$, ADM 40 mg/m$^2$, PSL 40 mg/m$^2$] on day 1, AMP [ADM 30 mg/m$^2$, MCNU 60 mg/m$^2$, PSL 40 mg/m$^2$] on day 8, and VECP [VDS 2.4 mg/m$^2$ on day 15, ETP 100 mg/m$^2$ on days 15–17, CBDCA 250 mg/m$^2$ on day15, PSL 40 mg/m$^2$ on days 15–17] on days 15–17, and the next course was to be started on day 29. The modifications in mLSG15 as compared to LSG15 were as follows: (1) The total number of cycles was reduced from 7 to 6 because of progressive cytopenia, especially thrombocytopenia, after repeating the VCAP-AMP-VECP therapy. (2) Cytarabine 40 mg was added to MTX 15 mg and PSL 10 mg for prophylactic intrathecal administration, at the recovery phases of courses 1, 3, and 5 because of the high frequency of central nervous system relapse in the JCOG9303 study. One hundred and eighteen patients were randomized. Seventy-two percent of the patients responded, with 23 patients achieving CR (40%) and 18 achieving PR (32%) in mLSG15. The ORR was 66%, with 15 patients achieving CR (25%) and 25 achieving PR (41%) in CHOP-14. The CR rate was higher in the mLSG15 arm than CHOP-14 arm (40% vs. 25%, respectively; $P = 0.020$). The median progression-free survival (PFS) time and PFS at 1 year in the former were 7.0 months and 28%, respectively, compared to 5.4 months and 16% in the latter ($P = 0.10$). The MST and OS at 3 years were, respectively, 12.7 months and 24% in the former and 10.9 months and 13% in the latter ($P = 0.085$). After the adjustment of patients' characteristics by Cox regression, the P value for OS became 0.029 because of unbalanced prognostic factors such as bulky lesions and B symptoms. In mLSG15 versus CHOP-14, the percentage with grade 4 neutropenia, percentage with grade 4 thrombocytopenia, and percentage with grade 3–4 infection were 98% versus 83%, 74% versus 17%, and 32% versus 15%, respectively. Three treatment-related deaths (TRDs), two from sepsis and one from interstitial pneumonitis related to neutropenia, were reported in the former. The longer OS at 3 years and higher CR rate with mLSG15 than CHOP-14 suggest mLSG15 to be a more effective regimen at the expense of greater toxicities providing a basis for future investigations in the treatment of ATL [2]. The superiority of VCAP-AMP-VECP in mLSG15 to CHOP-14 may be explained by the more prolonged, dose-dense schedule of therapy in addition to four more drugs. In addition, agents such as CBDCA and MCNU not affected by multidrug-resistance (MDR)-related genes, which were frequently expressed in ATL cells at onset, were incorporated [12]. Intrathecal prophylaxis, which was incorporated in both arms of the phase III study, should be considered for patients with aggressive ATL even in the absence of clinical symptoms because a previous analysis revealed that more than half of relapses at a new site after chemotherapy occurred in the CNS [13]. However, the prognosis of aggressive ATL after chemotherapy is still poor as compared to other hematological malignancies. Allo-HSCT is now recommended for the treatment of relatively young patients with aggressive ATL (refer to another chapter). To evaluate the efficacy of allo-HSCT, possibly associated with a graft-versus-ATL effect, more accurately, especially in view of a comparison with intensive chemotherapy, a prospective multicenter phase II study of mLSG15 chemotherapy followed by up-front allo-HSCT, comparing the results with historical control in JCOG9801, is ongoing (JCOG0907).

## 10.2 Development of Anti-CCR4 Antibody with Chemotherapy for Aggressive ATL

CC chemokine receptor 4 (CCR4) is expressed on normal T helper type 2 and regulatory T (Treg) cells and on certain types of T-cell neoplasms. CCR4 is expressed on the neoplastic cells of most ATL patients, and this expression has been associated with the cutaneous manifestation and poor prognosis [14]. The aberrant expression of Fra-2 promotes that of CCR4 and cell proliferation in ATL cells [15]. CCR4 mutation is frequently observed in ATL cells and associated with gain of function [16]. The defucosylated humanized anti-CCR4 monoclonal antibody (mogamulizumab), the ADCC activity of which was stronger than that of the usual Ab in preclinical analysis using primary ATL and effector cells, was approved for the treatment of relapsed/refractory ATL in Japan based on the results of phase I and II studies, with a response rate of approximately 50% and manageable toxicities including moderate to severe skin reactions for relapsed aggressive ATL [4, 17]. The findings of a subsequent randomized phase II study on intensive chemotherapy (mLSG15) +/− mogamulizumab for untreated aggressive ATL have recently been reported [18]. This combination was anticipated because the former was more effective for ATL cells in lymph nodes than those in the peripheral blood, while the opposite was true for the latter [2, 3]. The combination was well tolerated and produced a higher CR rate {52% (95% CI; 33, 71) vs. 33% (CI; 16, 55)}, respectively, with manageable hematological and cutaneous toxicities. Immunochemotherapy of mLSG15 + mogamulizumab is a promising and possible new standard therapy for aggressive ATL despite no difference in PFS and OS so far in relatively short observation period and small sample size.

## 10.3 Conclusion: Future of Multidisciplinary Treatment for ATL

IFN/AZT therapy is apparently promising for types with leukemic manifestation but not for lymphoma-type ATL, according to the retrospective meta-analysis from the USA, Europe, and Lebanon [19]. The results of a retrospective analysis in 73 patients with aggressive ATL (acute ATL, 29; lymphoma ATL, 44) suggested that chemotherapy with concurrent/sequential IFN/AZT as initial treatment might improve survival for both acute and lymphoma types of ATL compared with chemotherapy alone [20]. Further evaluation of IFN/AZT therapy alone or with chemotherapy or other modality including $As_2O_3$ is warranted in relation to subtypes of ATL.

Mogamulizumab eradicates Treg cells as well as ATL cells, and a preliminary retrospective analysis revealed that the agent with or without chemotherapy might increase the risk of acute GVHD and non-relapse mortality after allo-HSCT [21]. Further evaluation is warranted to establish the strategy of treatment of aggressive ATL in multidisciplinary treatment with mogamulizumab.

Chemotherapy of aggressive ATL has advanced in several decades with new cytotoxic agents, supportive cares including G-CSF and prophylaxis, and treatment of opportunistic infections and anti-CCR4 antibody. Several new molecular targeting, immune-regulatory agents and human T-cell leukemia virus type I (HTLV-1) vaccines are now under evaluation or in preparation for relapsed and/or refractory aggressive ATL. Then, among them, promising agents should be evaluated with chemotherapy for newly diagnosed aggressive ATL.

## References

1. Tsukasaki K, Hermine O, Bazarbachi A, Ratner L, Ramos JC, Harrington Jr W, et al. Definition, prognostic factors, treatment, and response criteria of adult T-cell leukemia-lymphoma: a proposal from an international consensus meeting. J Clin Oncol. 2009;27:453–9.
2. Tsukasaki K, Utsunomiya A, Fukuda H, Shibata T, Fukushima T, Takatsuka Y, et al. VCAP-AMP-VECP compared with biweekly CHOP for adult T-cell leukemia-lymphoma: Japan Clinical Oncology Group Study JCOG9801. J Clin Oncol. 2007;25:5458–64.

3. Ishida T, Joh T, Uike N, Yamamoto K, Utsunomiya A, Yoshida S, et al. Defucosylated anti-CCR4 monoclonal antibody (KW-0761) for relapsed adult T-cell leukemia-lymphoma: a multicenter phase II study. J Clin Oncol. 2012;30:837–42.
4. Tsukasaki K, Tobinai K, Hotta T, Shimoyama M. Lymphoma Study Group of JCOG. Jpn J Clin Oncol. 2012;42:85–95.
5. Vose J, Armitage J, Weisenburger D. International peripheral T-cell and natural killer/T-cell lymphoma study: pathology findings and clinical outcomes. J Clin Oncol. 2008;26 (25):4124–30.
6. Shimoyama M, Ichimaru M, Yunoki K, Oota K, Ogawa M. Final results of cooperative study of VEPA [vincristine, cyclophosphamide (endoxan), prednisolone and adriamycin] therapy in advanced adult non-Hodgkin's lymphoma: relation between T- or B-Cell phenotype and response. Jpn J Clin Oncol. 1982;12:227–37.
7. Shimoyama M, Ota K, Kikuchi M, Yunoki K, Konda S, Takatsuki K, et al. Chemotherapeutic results and prognostic factors of patients with advanced non-Hodgkin's lymphoma treated with VEPA or VEPA-M. J Clin Oncol. 1988;6:128–41.
8. Tobinai K, Shimoyama M, Minato K, Shirakawa S, Kobayashi T, Hotta T, et al. Japan Clinical Oncology Group phase II trial of second-generation 'LSG4 protocol' in aggressive T- and B-lymphoma: a new predictive model for T-and B-lymphoma. Proc Am Soc Clin Oncol. 1994;13:378a. (Abstract)
9. Tobinai K, Uike N, Saburi Y, et al. Phase II study of cladribine (2-chlorodeoxyadenosine) in relapsed or refractory adult T-cell leukemia-lymphoma. Int J Hematol. 2003;77:512–7.
10. Tsukasaki K, Tobinai K, Shimoyama M, Kozuru M, Uike N, Yamada Y, et al. Deoxycoformycin-containing combination chemotherapy for adult T-cell leukemia-lymphoma: Japan Clinical Oncology Group study (JCOG9109). Int J Hematol. 2003;77:164–70.
11. Yamada Y, Tomonaga M, Fukuda H, Hanada S, Utsunomiya A, Tara M, et al. A new G-CSF-supported combination chemotherapy, LSG15, for adult T-cell leukemia-lymphoma (ATL): Japan Clinical Oncology Group (JCOG) Study 9303. Br J Haematol. 2001;113:375–82.
12. Ohno N, Tani A, Uozumi K, et al. Expression of functional lung resistance–related protein predicts poor outcome in adult T-cell leukemia. Blood. 2001;98:1160–5.
13. Tsukasaki K, Ikeda S, Murata K, et al. Characteristics of chemotherapy-induced clinical remissionin long survivors with aggressive adult T-cell leukemia/lymphoma. Leuk Res. 1993;17:157–66.
14. Ishida T, Utsunomiya A, Iida S, Inagaki H, Takatsuka Y, Kusumoto S, et al. Clinical significance of CCR4 expression in adult T-cell leukemia/lymphoma: its close association with skin involvement and unfavorable outcome. Clin Cancer Res. 2003;9:3625–34.
15. Nakayama T, Hieshima K, Arao T, et al. Aberrant expression of Fra-2 promotes CCR4 expression and cell proliferation in adult T-cell leukemia. Oncogene. 2008;27:3221–32.
16. Nakagawa M, Schmitz R, Xiao W, et al. Gain-of-function CCR4 mutations in adult T cell leukemia/lymphoma. J Exp Med. 2014;211(13):2497–505.
17. Yamamoto K, Utsunomiya A, Tobinai K, Tsukasaki K, Uike N, Uozumi K, et al. Phase I study of KW-0761, a defucosylated humanized anti-CCR4 antibody, in relapsed patients with adult T-cell leukemia-lymphoma and peripheral T-cell lymphoma. J Clin Oncol. 2010;28:1591–8.
18. Ishida T, Jo T, Takemoto S, et al. Dose-intensified chemotherapy alone or in combination with mogamulizumab in newly diagnosed aggressive adult T-cell leukaemia-lymphoma: a randomized phase II study. Br J Haematol. 2015;169(5):672–82.
19. Bazarbachi A, Plumelle Y, Ramos JC, Tortevoye P, Otrock Z, Taylor G, et al. Meta-analysis on the use of zidovudine and interferon-alfa in adult T-cell leukemia/lymphoma showing improved survival in the leukemic subtypes. J Clin Oncol. 2010;27:417–23.
20. Hodson A, Crichton S, Montoto S, et al. Use of zidovudine and interferon alfa with chemotherapy improves survival in both acute and lymphoma subtypes of adult T-cell leukemia/lymphoma. J Clin Oncol. 2011;29(35):4696–701.
21. Inoue Y, Fuji S, Tanosaki R, Fukuda T. Pretransplant mogamulizumab against ATLL might increase the risk of acute GVHD and non-relapse mortality. Bone Marrow Transplant. 2016 May;51(5):725–7.

# Chapter 11
# Transplantation for Aggressive Adult T-Cell Leukemia/Lymphoma (ATL)

**Atae Utsunomiya**

## 11.1 Introduction

Adult T-cell leukemia-lymphoma (ATL) is an intractable disease caused by human T-cell leukemia virus type I (HTLV-1) [1–3]. The median overall survival (OS) time for patients with aggressive-type ATL is only about 1 year; new therapeutic strategies are required for these patients [4, 5].

At the present time, allogeneic hematopoietic stem cell transplantation (allo-HSCT) is considered to be the only curative treatment for ATL patients [6]. However, the efficacy of this therapy is limited by high transplant-related mortality (TRM) and relapse rates. Herein, a review of allo-HSCT for the treatment of aggressive-type ATL in the past, present, and future is presented.

## 11.2 History of HSCT

It has been reported that ATL cells are resistant to chemotherapeutic agents due to the expression of multidrug resistance genes [7, 8]. In order to overcome this drug resistance, autologous bone marrow transplantation (auto-BMT) with high-dose chemotherapeutic agents was undertaken and reported by Asou et al. in a case in 1985 [9]. However, the OS time was not prolonged because of early relapse in this case. Since that report, several cases of autologous HSCT (auto-HSCT) have been reported, but improved OS times were not obtained in these cases because of early relapse or infections [10].

A. Utsunomiya (✉)
Department of Hematology, Imamura Bun-in Hospital, 11-23 Kamoikeshinmachi, Kagoshima 890-0064, Japan
e-mail: autsunomiya@jiaikai.jp



T. Watanabe, T. Fukushima (eds.), *Adult T-cell Leukemia/Lymphoma*,
DOI 10.1007/978-4-431-56523-9_11

On the other hand, Sobue et al. first reported a case of allogeneic BMT (allo-BMT) for a patient with aggressive ATL in 1987. The patient appeared to have had been successfully treated with allo-BMT, but died of interstitial pneumonitis due to cytomegalovirus infection 205 days after the transplantation [11]. Subsequently, several ATL cases have been successfully treated with allo-HSCT. We reported ten ATL cases treated with allo-HSCT in 2001, concluding that allo-HSCT might improve the prognoses of ATL patients [12].

Since our report, the number of ATL patients receiving allo-HSCT has been increasing over time [13]; between 1991 and 2013, 1,535 ATL cases were reported to have received allo-HSCT, and approximately 150 ATL patients are now receiving allo-HSCT annually [13].

## 11.3 Transplant Procedure

There are two transplant procedures: auto-HSCT and allo-HSCT. Conditioning regimens consist of myeloablative conditioning (MAC) and reduced-intensity conditioning (RIC) [14, 15]. Three stem cell sources, bone marrow (BM), peripheral blood stem cells (PBSC), and cord blood (CB), are used from the patient, a related donor or an unrelated donor. All transplant procedures are used for ATL patients except for auto-HSCT, which does not improve the OS time because of early relapse or infectious complications [10].

## 11.4 Prognostic Factors

Five prognostic factors have been associated with a poor prognosis in a study by the Japan Clinical Oncology Group-Lymphoma Study Group (JCOG-LSG). These include poor performance status (PS), high serum lactate dehydrogenase (LDH), over 40 years of age, total number of involved lesions, and hypercalcemia [16]. Multivariate analysis revealed other poor prognostic factors, including eosinophilia, thrombocytopenia, bone marrow invasion, high serum interleukin-5, expression of CC chemokine receptor 4 (CCR4), lung resistance protein, *P53* mutation, and *P16* deletion [17, 18]. Recently, Katsuya et al. have identified five poor prognostic factors, i.e., advanced Ann Arbor stage, poor Eastern Cooperative Oncology Group PS, the increased age, decrease in serum albumin, and elevated soluble interleukin-2 receptor (sIL-2R), and they reported that the prognoses differ among three groups (low, intermediate, and high risk) stratified by a combination of these prognostic factors [19]. On the other hand, four factors, i.e., age over 40 years, male sex, non-complete remission (non-CR), and cord blood transplantation (CBT), have been reported to influence the OS time of patients who received allo-HSCT in a nationwide retrospective study [20]. In univariate analysis, an elevated serum sIL-2R level has been identified as a poor prognostic factor at both the time of diagnosis and the time of preconditioning [21, 22]. In addition, the European Group for Blood and Marrow Transplantation (EBMT) risk score and elevated sIL-2R are significant poor prognostic factors, and they can be used in combination to stratify patients into three risk groups (low, intermediate, and high risk) [23].

## 11.5 Results of Allo-HSCT

The outcomes of allo-HSCT for patients with aggressive ATL are shown in Table 11.1 [5]. Although the prognoses of ATL patients were improved with allo-HSCT, a high TRM rate using MAC remains one of the most important issues [5, 6]. In order to reduce the high TRM rate, reduced-intensity stem cell transplantation (RIST) has been applied for elderly ATL patients.

## 11.6 Results of Allo-HSCT According to the Intensity of Conditioning

The 3-year OS rate with a MAC or RIC regimen was 27–73% (Table 11.1) [5]. Since Okamura et al. first reported the feasibility of RIST for elderly ATL patients [24], a RIC regimen has been used more frequently for allo-HSCT in elderly ATL patients. No statistical differences were observed in the OS rates between patients receiving MAC and RIC regimens in a nationwide retrospective analysis [25]. The TRM rate was high with the MAC regimen, while it was low with RIC. On the other hand, there was a trend toward increased ATL-related deaths with RIC than with MAC [25].

## 11.7 Results of Allo-HSCT According to Stem Cell Source

There was no difference in the OS time between patients receiving BM cells and those receiving PBSC. A nationwide retrospective study revealed that the 3-year OS rate with BM cells or PBSC from HLA-matched related donors was 41%, while that with BM cells from HLA-matched unrelated donors was 39%. The 3-year OS rate using BM cells or PBSC from HLA-mismatched donors is 24%, while that using CB cells is 17% [20]. Thus, the OS rate of CBT was poorer than those of other transplant procedures [20]. It is thought that this poor outcome might be an effect of the increased patient age and/or poor disease condition. It has recently been reported that the OS rate of ATL patients undergoing CBT with a good disease status is improving [26, 27].

**Table 11.1** Summary of published reports on allogeneic hematopoietic stem cell transplantation in adult T-cell leukemia-lymphoma (ATL)

| Reference | Pt. No. | Median age (range) | Sex M/F | Subtype | Donor | Donor HTLV-1 Ab | Stem cell source | Disease status at SCT | Conditioning regimen | Cause of death | Outcome |
|---|---|---|---|---|---|---|---|---|---|---|---|
| Utsunomiya (BMT, 2001) | 10 | 45 | 7/3 | Acute:8 | MSD:9 | Neg:7 | BM:8 | CR:4 | MAC:10 | TRM:4 | Median leukemia-free survival 17.5 + M (range 3.7–34.4+) |
| | | | | Lymphoma:1 | | | PB:1 | PR:5 | | | |
| | | (33–51) | | Other:1 | MUD:1 | Posi:3 | BM + PB:1 | NR:1 | | | |
| Kami (BJH, 2003) | 11 | 47 | 7/4 | Acute:5 | MSD:9 | Neg:9 | BM:7 | CR:6 | MAC:9 | TRM:7 | 1Y–OS |
| | | | | Lymphoma:4 | PMRD:1 | | PB:3 | PR:1 | RIC:2 | | |
| | | (15–59) | | Other:2 | MUD:1 | Posi:2 | BM + PB:1 | PD:4 | | | 54.5 ± 30.0% |
| Fukushima (Leukemia, 2005) | 40 | 44 | 22/18 | Acute:30 | MSD:27 | Neg:27 | BM:21 | CR:15 | MAC: most cases | TRM:16 | 3Y-0S |
| | | | | Lymphoma:10 | PMRD:5 | Posi:9 | | PR:13 | | Unk:1 | |
| | | (28–53) | | | NUD:8 | NE:4 | PB:19 | NC:3 | | ATL:4 | 45.3% |
| | | | | | | | | PD:9 | | | |
| Kato (BBMT, 2007) | 33 | 49 | 18/15 | Acute:20 | MUD:33 | Neg:33 | BM:33 | CR + PR:15 | MAC:27 | TRM:9 | 1Y–OS |
| | | | | Lymphoma:7 | | | | NR:14 | | ATL:2 | |
| | | (24–59) | | NE:6 | | | | NE:4 | RIC:6 | NE:3 | 49.5% |
| Shiratori (BBMT, 2008) | 15 | 57 | 3/12 | Acute:6 | MSD:10 | Neg:13 | BM:8 | CR:9 | MAC:5 | TRM:2 | 3Y–OS |
| | | | | Lymphoma:8 | | | PB:4 | PR:5 | | | |
| | | (41–66) | | Others:1 | MRD:5 | Posi:2 | BM + PB:3 | PD:1 | RIC:10 | ATL:2 | 73.3% |
| Nakase (BMT, 2006) | 8 | 49 | 2/6 | Acute:5 | MUD:3 | Neg:8 | BM:8 | CR:6 | MAC:5 | TRM:2 | Median OS 20 M (range 0–43) |
| | | (45–59) | | Lymphoma:3 | PMUD:5 | | | nonCR:2 | RIC:3 | ATL:1 | |
| Nakamura (IJH, 2012) | 10 | 51 | 6/4 | Acute:9 | PMUD:10 | Neg: 10 | UCB | CR:2 | MAC:6 | ATL:4 | 2Y–OS:40% |
| | | | | | | | | PR:4 | | Sepsis:1 | |
| | | (31–64) | | Lymphoma:1 | | | | SD:1 | RIC:4 | GVHD + ATL:1 | (95% CI 67–12) |
| | | | | | | | | PD:3 | | | |

| | | | | | | | | | | | |
|---|---|---|---|---|---|---|---|---|---|---|---|
| Fukushima (IJH, 2013) | 27 | 52 | 18/9 | Acute:17 | MUD:1 | Neg:27 | UCB | CR:5 | MAC:9 | TRM:10 | 3Y–OS:27.4% |
| | | | | | | | | PR:11 | | | |
| | | (41–63) | | Lymphoma:10 | PMUD:26 | | | PIF:5 | RIC:18 | ATL:9 | |
| | | | | | | | | REL:6 | | | |
| Bazarbachi (BMT, 2014) | 17 | 47 | 9/8 | Acute:5 | MSD:6 | ND | ND | CR:9 | MAC:4 | ATL:8 | 3Y–OS:34.3% |
| | | | | Lymphoma:10 | MUD:7 | | | PR:4 | | GVHD:2 | |
| | | | | Chro/Smold:2 | UnK:1 | | | PD:4 | RIC:13 | Sepsis:1 | |
| | | (21–58) | | | PMRD:3 | | | | | | |

*ATL* adult T-cell leukemia-lymphoma, *BBMT* biology of blood and marrow transplantation, *BJH British Journal of Haematology*, *BMT* bone marrow transplantation, *Chro/Smold* chronic/smoldering, *CR* complete remission, *GVHD* graft-versus-host disease, *IJH International Journal of Hematology*, *M* month, *MAC* myeloablative conditioning, *MSD* HLA-matched sibling donor, *MUD* HLA-matched unrelated donor, *NC* no change, *ND* not described, *NE* not evaluable, *Neg* negative, *NR* no response, *OS* overall survival, *PD* progressive disease, *PIF* primary induction failure, *Posi* positive, *PMRD* HLA partially matched related donor, *PMUD* HLA partially matched unrelated donor, *PR* partial remission, *REL* refractory after relapse, *RIC* reduced-intensity conditioning, *SCT* stem cell transplantation, *SD* stable disease, *TRM* transplant-related mortality, *UCB* unrelated cord blood, *UnK* unknown

## 11.8 Timing of Allo-HSCT

It has been reported that the outcomes of ATL patients receiving allo-HSCT in CR are better than those in non-CR [20]. We have also reported that the OS rate of patients who received allo-HSCT from a related donor within 100 days after the establishment of their ATL diagnosis was better than that of patients waiting more than 100 days after diagnosis [28]. Interestingly, this effect was also observed in non-CR patients [28]. These findings suggest that many courses of chemotherapy might induce a poor condition in ATL patients, and a poor PS might result in poor patient outcomes after transplantation.

## 11.9 Minimum Residual Disease

The quantification of HTLV-1 proviral loads in peripheral blood (PB) is very useful for the early detection of leukemic ATL relapse after allo-HSCT. HTLV-1, however, exists not only in ATL cells but also in the recipient's non-ATL cells. In addition, if patients receive allo-HSCT from HTLV-1 carrier donors, HTLV-1 will be transferred from the donor to the recipient. Furthermore, non-HTLV-1-infected donor cells can be infected by HTLV-1 from ATL cells or HTLV-1-infected non-ATL cells of recipient origin. Thus, these four types of HTLV-1-infected cells exist in PB (Fig. 11.1); this principle has been clearly demonstrated by Yamasaki et al. [29].

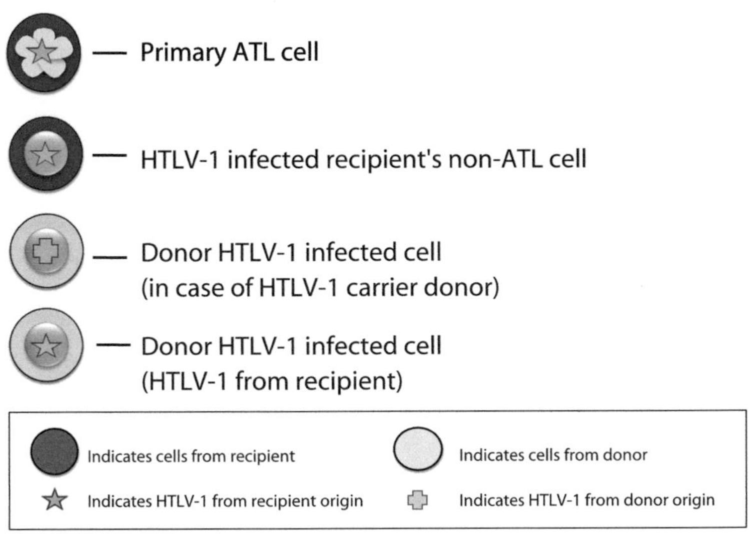


**Fig. 11.1** HTLV-1-infected cells after allo-HSCT. HTLV-1-infected cells after allo-HSCT include four types of cells: primary ATL cells, the HTLV-1-infected recipient's non-ATL cells, donor HTLV-1 -infected cells in the case of patients who received an allo-HSCT from an HTLV-1 carrier donor, and donor HTLV-1-infected cells that have been infected with HTLV-1 from recipients after allo-HSCT

It has been reported that the number of HTLV-1-infected cells decreases shortly after allo-HSCT, but HTLV-1-negative donor cells are sometimes infected by HTLV-1 1 or 2 years after allo-HSCT [30]. Although the monitoring of HTLV-1 proviral loads is useful for leukemic relapse, it should be considered that HTLV-1-infected cells do not necessarily represent only ATL cells of the recipient.

## 11.10 Graft-Versus-ATL Effect

We have reported that the cessation of immunosuppressants and/or donor lymphocyte infusion (DLI) induced another remission in relapsed ATL patients after allo-HSCT [31]; this phenomenon is thought to be caused by a graft-versus-ATL (Gv-ATL) effect. Harashima et al. reported that Tax-specific cytotoxic T lymphocytes played an important role in these Gv-ATL effects [32].

It has been recently reported that although chemotherapy or DLI alone did not induce remission in relapsed ATL patients after allo-HSCT, DLI after the reduction of tumor burden with chemotherapy effectively induced remission [33]. These phenomena might indicate that the reduction of tumor size plays a crucial role in the induction of the Gv-ATL effect.

## 11.11 Role of Mogamulizumab

A humanized anti-CCR4 monoclonal antibody, mogamulizumab, has been approved as a new molecular targeting drug for ATL patients [34]. Single agent of mogamulizumab showed high efficacy for relapsed or refractory ATL [34], and a combination of VCAP-AMP-VECP (vincristine, cyclophosphamide, adriamycin, prednisone–adriamycin, ranimustine, prednisone–vindesine, etoposide, carboplatin, prednisone) therapy (modified LSG15 regimen) and mogamulizumab showed a 52% CR rate in newly diagnosed ATL patients [35]. Mogamulizumab is now used for ATL to improve the CR rate because the outcomes of ATL patients who received allo-HSCT are better than those in non-CR [20]. However, mogamulizumab can reduce not only ATL cells but also normal regulatory T cells [34, 35], which have critical roles in the control of acute graft-versus-host disease (GVHD). Actually, it has been reported that the administration of mogamulizumab before allo-HSCT increased non-relapse mortality and acute GVHD in ATL patients [36]. Therefore, we should use mogamulizumab appropriately, not only before conditioning but also after ATL relapse (Fig. 11.2).

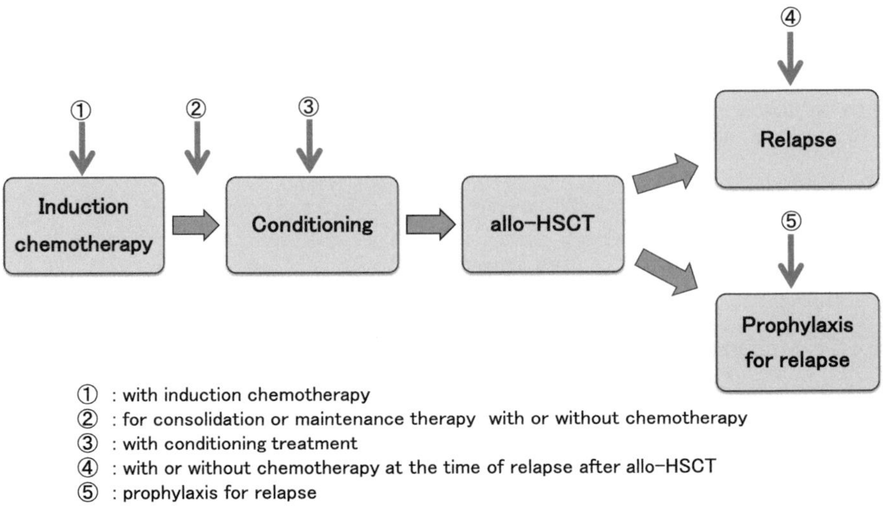


**Fig. 11.2** Mogamulizumab therapy for ATL patients receiving allo-HSCT. There are several timings in administration of mogamulizumab as shown in Fig. 11.2 (①–⑤). Since mogamulizumab can reduce not only ATL cells but also normal regulatory T-cells, which have critical roles in graft-versus-host disease, we do not recommend the administration of mogamulizumab as conditioning treatment

## 11.12 Donor Cell-Derived ATL

Donor cell-derived leukemia (DCL) has rarely been reported in patients with allo-HSCT [37]. Although the mechanism of the occurrence of DCL has not been elucidated, there are several possibilities, such as the existence of occult leukemia in donor cells or aberrant BM microenvironment in the recipients [37]. Three cases of DCL after allo-HSCT in ATL patients have been reported [38–40]. One had acute myeloid leukemia [38], and the other two had ATL [39, 40]. Both of the ATL patients had received allo-HSCT from HTLV-1 carriers [39, 40]. We should pay special attention to not only the relapse of ATL but also donor cell-derived ATL.

## 11.13 Indication for Allo-HSCT

The indication for allo-HSCT for ATL patients is the same as that for other hematological malignancies. The patient's age, disease status, PS, organ function, existence of active infection, and appropriate stem cell source are the main factors in deciding whether to perform allo-HSCT. In ATL patients, the inclusion criteria for allo-HSCT are as follows: ≤70 years of age (≤65 years of age if the patient receives allo-HSCT from an unrelated donor or CB), good disease status [CR, partial remission (PR) or stable disease (SD)], good performance status (PS = 0 or 1), and no active infection. Allo-HSCT is recommended to be performed within 6 months after the establishment of a diagnosis, if possible, because the OS time if it is performed more than 100 days from diagnosis is shorter than that if the patient is less than 100 days from the diagnosis in the patients who received allo-HSCT from related donors [28].

## 11.14 Eligibility of Donor

The eligibility criteria of donors for allo-HSCT in ATL patients are the same as those for other diseases, except for HTLV-1 carrier donors; in unrelated HSCT or in allo-HSCT for diseases other than ATL, HTLV-1 carriers are always excluded as donors. However, the eligibility of HTLV-1 carriers as related donors for ATL patients who receive allo-HSCT has not been determined. As donor cell-derived ATL after allo-HSCT using HTLV-1 carrier donors in ATL patients has been reported, we have to carefully determine the eligibility of HTLV-1 carriers for donors. Therefore, we examined the HTLV-1 status in detail by evaluating HTLV-1 proviral DNA in PB with not only Southern blot analysis but also real-time PCR. If the monoclonal or oligoclonal integration of HTLV-1 provirus has been detected in HTLV-1 carriers, these donors should be excluded.

Several HTLV-1 carrier recipients who had received a renal or liver transplantation developed ATL, probably due to the administration of immunosuppressants [41, 42]. Importantly, donor cell-derived ATL can occur in ATL patients because the recipients receive intensive immunosuppressive therapy after allo-HSCT. In allo-HSCT from HTLV-1 carrier donors, donor eligibility should be determined carefully based on the results of their HTLV-1 status. The copy number of HTLV-1 proviral loads, as determined with real-time PCR, is preferably $\leq$4 copies/100 PBMCs, without monoclonal or oligoclonal proliferation of HTLV-1, because high proviral loads in PB (>4 copies/100 PBMCs) have been reported as one of the risk factors for ATL development [43].

## 11.15 Future Directions

At the present time, the relapse rate of ATL after allo-HSCT increases when we attempt to reduce the TRM rate. In contrast, the TRM rate increases if we attempt to reduce the ATL relapse rate. The evaluation of new molecular targeting therapy and immunotherapy is underway [34, 35, 44–46]. In the near future, a combination of chemotherapy, allo-HSCT, molecular targeting therapy, and immunotherapy may bring promising outcomes for ATL patients.

## 11.16 Conclusions

Although some ATL patients can now be cured with allo-HSCT, the cure rate of ATL patients is still low due to the high TRM rate and frequent ATL relapse after allo-HSCT. The establishment of allo-HSCT with a high cure rate through the combination of new therapies is required for ATL therapy.

**Acknowledgment** This work was supported in part by the Practical Research for Innovative Cancer Control from Japan Agency for Medical Research and Development, AMED.

## References

1. Uchiyama T, Yodoi J, Sagawa K, Takatsuki K, Uchino H. Adult T-cell leukemia: clinical and hematologic features of 16 cases. Blood. 1977;50:481–92.
2. Poiesz BJ, Ruscetti FW, Gazdar AF, et al. Detection and isolation of type C retrovirus particles from fresh and cultured lymphocytes of a patient with cutaneous T-cell lymphoma. Proc Natl Acad Sci U S A. 1980;77:7415–9.
3. Hinuma Y, Nagata K, Hanaoka M, et al. Adult T-cell leukemia: antigen in an ATL cell line and detection of antibodies to the antigen in human sera. Proc Natl Acad Sci U S A. 1981;78:6476–80.
4. Ishitsuka K, Tamura K. Human T-cell leukaemia virus type I and adult T-cell leukaemia-lymphoma. Lancet Oncol. 2014;15:e517–26.
5. Utsunomiya A, Choi I, Chihara D, Seto M. Recent advances in treatment of adult T-cell leukemia-lymphomas. Cancer Sci. 2015;106:344–51.
6. Utsunomiya A, Nakano N, Takatsuka Y. Recent advances in allogeneic hematopoietic stem cell transplantation for adult T-cell leukemia-lymphoma. J Hematopoietic Cell Transplant. 2015;4:1–8.
7. Kuwazuru Y, Hanada S, Furukawa T, et al. Expression of P-glycoprotein in adult T-cell leukemia cells. Blood. 1990;76:2065–71.
8. Ohno N, Tani A, Uozumi K, et al. Expression of functional lung resistance-related protein predicts poor outcome in adult T-cell leukemia. Blood. 2001;98:1160–5.
9. Asou N, Sakai K, Yamaguchi K, et al. Autologous bone marrow transplantation in a patient with lymphoma type adult T cell leukemia. Rinshoketsueki. 1985;26:229–33.
10. Tsukasaki K, Maeda T, Arimura K, et al. Poor outcome of autologous stem cell transplantation for adult T cell leukemia/lymphoma: a case report and review of the literature. Bone Marrow Transplant. 1999;23:87–9.
11. Sobue R, Yamauchim T, Miyamura K, et al. Treatment of adult T cell leukemia with mega-dose cyclophosphamide and total body irradiation followed by allogeneic bone marrow transplantation. Bone Marrow Transplant. 1987;2:441–4.
12. Utsunomiya A, Miyazaki Y, Takatsuka Y, et al. Improved outcome of adult T cell leukemia/lymphoma with allogeneic hematopoietic stem cell transplantation. Bone Marrow Transplant. 2001;27:15–20.
13. Hematopoietic Cell Transplantation in Japan. Annual Report of Nationwide Survey 2014. The Japanese Data Center for Hematopoietic Cell Transplantation/The Japan Society for Hematopoietic Cell Transplantation 2015, March 15, 2015.
14. Giralt S, Ballen K, Rizzo D, et al. Reduced-intensity conditioning regimen workshop: defining the dose spectrum. Report of a workshop convened by the center for international blood and marrow transplant research. Biol Blood Marrow Transplant. 2009;15:367–9.

15. Bacigalupo A, Ballen K, Rizzo D, et al. Defining the intensity of conditioning regimens: working definitions. Biol Blood Marrow Transplant. 2009;15:1628–33.
16. LYMPHOMA STUDY GROUP (1984–1987). Major prognostic factors of patients with adult T-cell leukemia-lymphoma: a cooperative study. Leuk Res. 1991;15:81–90.
17. Utsunomiya A, Ishida T, Inagaki A, et al. Clinical significance of a blood eosinophilia in adult T-cell leukemia/lymphoma: a blood eosinophilia is a significant unfavorable prognostic factor. Leuk Res. 2007;31:915–20.
18. Tsukasaki K, Tobinai K. Clinical trials and treatment of ATL. Leuk Res Treat. 2012;2012:101754.
19. Katsuya H, Yamanaka T, Ishitsuka K, et al. Prognostic index for acute- and lymphoma-type adult T-cell leukemia/lymphoma. J Clin Oncol. 2012;30:1635–40.
20. Hishizawa M, Kanda J, Utsunomiya A, et al. Transplantation of allogeneic hematopoietic stem cells for adult T-cell leukemia: a nationwide retrospective study. Blood. 2011;116:1369–76.
21. Shigematsu A, Kobayashi N, Yasui H, et al. High level of serum soluble interleukin-2 receptor at transplantation predicts poor outcome of allogeneic stem cell transplantation for adult T cell leukemia. Biol Blood Marrow Transplant. 2014;20:801–5.
22. Kawada H, Yoshimitsu M, Nakamura D, et al. A retrospective analysis of treatment outcomes in adult T cell leukemia/lymphoma patients with aggressive disease treated with or without allogeneic stem cell transplantation: a single-center experience. Biol Blood Marrow Transplant. 2015;21:696–700.
23. Tokunaga M, Uto H, Takeuchi S, et al. Newly identified poor prognostic factors for adult T-cell leukemia-lymphoma treated with allogeneic hematopoietic stem cell transplantation. Leuk Lymhoma. 2017; 58: 37–44.
24. Okamura J, Utsunomiya A, Tanosaki R, et al. Allogeneic stem-cell transplantation with reduced conditioning intensity as a novel immunotherapy and antiviral therapy for adult T-cell leukemia/lymphoma. Blood. 2005;105:4143–5.
25. Ishida T, Hishizawa M, Kato K, et al. Allogeneic hematopoietic stem cell transplantation for adult T-cell leukemia-lymphoma with special emphasis on preconditioning regimen: a nationwide retrospective study. Blood. 2012;120:1734–41.
26. Nakamura T, Oku E, Nomura K, et al. Unrelated cord blood transplantation for patients with adult T-cell leukemia/lymphoma: experience at a single institute. Int J Hematol. 2012;96:657–63.
27. Fukushima T, Itonaga H, Moriuchi Y, et al. Feasibility of cord blood transplantation in chemosensitive adult T-cell leukemia/lymphoma: a retrospective analysis of the Nagasaki Transplantation Network. Int J Hematol. 2013;97:485–90.
28. Fuji S, Fujiwara H, Nakano N, et al. Early application of related SCT might improve clinical outcome in adult T-cell leukemia/lymphoma. Bone Marrow Transplant. 2016; 51: 205–11.
29. Yamasaki R, Miyazaki Y, Moriuchi Y, et al. Small number of HTLV-1-positive cells frequently remains during complete remission after allogeneic hematopoietic stem cell transplantation that are heterogeneous in origin among cases with adult T-cell leukemia/lymphoma. Leukemia. 2007;21:1212–7.
30. Choi I, Tanosaki R, Uike N, et al. Long-term outcomes after hematopoietic SCT for adult T-cell leukemia/lymphoma: results of prospective trials. Bone Marrow Transplant. 2011;46:116–8.
31. Yonekura K, Utsunomiya A, Takatsuka Y, et al. Graft-versus-adult T-cell leukemia/lymphoma effect following allogeneic hematopoietic stem cell transplantation. Bone Marrow Transplant. 2008;41:1029–35.
32. Harashima N, Kurihara K, Utsunomiya A, et al. Graft-versus-Tax response in adult T-cell leukemia patients after hematopoietic stem cell transplantation. Cancer Res. 2004;64:391–9.
33. Itonaga H, Tsushima H, Taguchi J, et al. Treatment of relapsed adult T-cell leukemia/lymphoma after allogeneic hematopoietic stem cell transplantation: the Nagasaki Transplant Group experience. Blood. 2013;121:219–25.

34. Ishida T, Joh T, Uike N, et al. Defucosylated anti-CCR4 monoclonal antibody (KW-0761) for relapsed adult T-cell leukemia-lymphoma: a multicenter phase II study. J Clin Oncol. 2012;30:837–42.
35. Ishida T, Jo T, Takemoto S, et al. Dose-intensified chemotherapy alone or in combination with mogamulizumab in newly diagnosed aggressive adult T-cell leukaemia-lymphoma: a randomized phase II study. Br J Haematol. 2015;169:672–82.
36. Fuji S, Inoue Y, Utsunomiya A, et al. Pretransplantation anti-CCR4 antibody mogamulizumab against adult T-cell leukemia/lymphoma is associated with significantly increased risks of severe and corticosteroid-refractory graft-versus-host disease, nonrelapse mortality, and overall mortality. J Clin Oncol. 2016; 34: 3426–33.
37. Wiseman DH. Donor cell leukemia: a review. Biol Blood Marrow Transplant. 2011;17:771–89.
38. Matsunaga T, Murase K, Yoshida M, et al. Donor cell derived myeloid leukemia after allogeneic cord blood transplantation in a patient with adult T-cell lymphoma. Am J Hematol. 2005;79:294–8.
39. Tamaki H, Matsuoka M. Donor-derived T-cell leukemia after bone marrow transplantation. New Engl J Med. 2006;354:1758–9.
40. Nakamizo A, Akagi Y, Amano T, et al. Donor-derived adult T-cell leukaemia. Lancet. 2011;377:1124.
41. Hoshida Y, Li T, Dong Z, et al. Lymphoproliferative disorders in renal transplant patients in Japan. Int J Cancer. 2001;91:869–75.
42. Yoshizumi T, Shirabe K, Ikegami T, et al. Impact of human T cell leukemia virus type 1 in living donor liver transplantation. Am J Transplant. 2012;12:1479–85.
43. Iwanaga M, Watanabe T, Utsunomiya A, et al. Human T-cell leukemia virus type I (HTLV-1) proviral load and disease progression in asymptomatic HTLV-1 carriers. Blood. 2010;116:1211–9.
44. Kozako T, Yoshimitsu M, Fujiwara H, et al. PD-1/PD-L1 expression in human T-cell leukemia virus type 1 carriers and adult T-cell leukemia/lymphoma patients. Leukemia. 2009;23:375–82.
45. Nishikawa H, Maeda Y, Ishida T, et al. Cancer/testis antigens are novel targets of immunotherapy for adult T-cell leukemia/lymphoma. Blood. 2012;119:3097–104.
46. Suehiro Y, Hasegawa A, Iino T, et al. Clinical outcomes of a novel therapeutic vaccine with Tax peptide-pulsed dendritic cells for adult T cell leukaemia/lymphoma in a pilot study. Br J Haematol. 2015;169:356–67.

# Chapter 12
# New Agents of Adult T-cell Leukemia/ Lymphoma (ATL)

**Wataru Munakata and Kensei Tobinai**

## 12.1 Introduction

Adult T-cell leukemia-lymphoma (ATL) is a distinct subtype of peripheral T-cell lymphomas (PTCLs) caused by human T-cell leukemia virus type I (HTLV-1) and is relatively frequent in southwestern Japan, West Africa, the Caribbean islands, and Brazil, which are HTLV-1 endemic areas [1, 2]. ATL is clinically classified into four disease subtypes (acute, lymphoma, chronic, and smoldering), based on clinical features including leukemic changes, high lactate dehydrogenase, hypercalcemia, and organ infiltration, and it was reported that the median survival time varies according to the disease type: acute type, 6 months; lymphoma type, 10 months; chronic type, 24 months; and smoldering type, 3 years or more [3]. It is recommended that treatment strategies should be selected according to the disease subtype [3]. In Japan, the acute type, lymphoma type, and chronic type with unfavorable prognostic factors have been regarded as aggressive ATL subtypes requiring immediate treatment. Generally, the disease is resistant to conventional chemotherapeutic agents in most ATL patients, and limited treatment options currently exist; thus, ATL of these aggressive forms has the worst prognosis among various major subtypes of PTCL, with 5-year overall survival (OS) and failure-free survival (FFS) rates of 14% and 12%, respectively [4]. A phase III trial for previously untreated patients with aggressive ATL (acute, lymphoma, or unfavorable chronic type) revealed that a dose-intensified multidrug regimen (modified LSG15), VCAP-AMP-VECP (vincristine, cyclophosphamide, doxorubicin, and prednisone; doxorubicin, ranimustine, and prednisone; and vindesine, etoposide, carboplatin, and prednisone), resulted in median progression-free survival (PFS)

W. Munakata (✉) • K. Tobinai
Department of Hematology, National Cancer Center Hospital, 5-1-1Tsukiji, Chuo-ku, Tokyo 104-0045, Japan
e-mail: wmunakat@ncc.go.jp; ktobinai@ncc.go.jp



T. Watanabe, T. Fukushima (eds.), *Adult T-cell Leukemia/Lymphoma*,
DOI 10.1007/978-4-431-56523-9_12

**Table 12.1** Novel agents for ATL

| | Mogamulizumab monotherapy [22] | Mogamulizumab + VCAP-AMP-VECP [23] | Lenalidomide monotherapy [35] | Brentuximab vedotin + CHP [38] |
|---|---|---|---|---|
| Number | 26 relapsed ATL | 29 untreated ATL | 9 relapsed ATL | 2 untreated ATL |
| Treatment | Weekly × 8 doses | 4 cycles of VCAP-AMP-VECP + 8 doses once every 2 weeks | Daily | Once every 3 weeks for 6 cycles |
| ORR (%) | 50% (13/26) | 86% (25/29) | 33% (3/9) | 100% (2/2) |
| CR (%) | 31% (8/26) | 52% (15/29) | 0% (0/9) | 100% (2/2) |

*CR* complete response, *ORR* overall response rate

and OS of 7.0 and 12.7 months, respectively, which were superior to those of the comparator arm, CHOP-14 [5]. However, since the outcome achieved by this dose-intensified regimen was still inferior to that in other PTCLs and B-cell non-Hodgkin lymphomas, further improvements were deemed necessary. Allogeneic hematopoietic stem-cell transplantation has evolved into a promising approach in treating patients with ATL over the last decade. However, only a small fraction of patients with ATL can benefit from transplantation [6–8]. Therefore, the development of alternative treatment strategies or effective novel drugs for patients with ATL, especially for elderly or frail patients who are ineligible for allogeneic hematopoietic stem-cell transplantation or intensive chemotherapy, is an urgent issue. In this chapter, we will discuss the novel drugs for ATL (Table 12.1).

## 12.2 CC Chemokine Receptor 4 (CCR4) and Mogamulizumab

Chemokines, which are a small family of cytokines, act as signaling molecules in the migration and tissue homing of various leukocytes. Among them, thymus- and activation-regulated chemokine (TARC) and monocyte-derived chemokine (MDC) induce the selective recruitment of distinct subsets of T cells by triggering the chemokine receptor, CCR4. CCR4 is a seven-transmembrane G-protein-coupled receptor that is a marker for type 2 helper T cells (Th2) and regulatory T (Treg) cells [9, 10]. Although the expression of CCR4 on normal cells such as Th2 cells can be partly regulated by the ligand [11], especially MDC, this regulation by ligands on tumor cells has not yet been fully elucidated. Ishida et al. examined ATL cells obtained from 103 patients with ATL and found that tumor cells from approximately 90% of patients were positive for the expression of CCR4 [12] (Table 12.2). They also showed that patients with CCR4-positive ATL were more likely to have skin infiltration and a worse outcome than those with CCR4-negative ATL, which indicated that CCR4 played an important pathogenetic role in ATL [12]. CCR4 is also expressed on tumor cells in approximately 30–65% of patients with other types

**Table 12.2** CCR4 expression in mature T-cell and NK-cell neoplasms [12–14]

| Pathological subtypes | Positivity | |
|---|---|---|
| NK-/T-cell lymphoma, nasal type | 1/27 | (4%) |
| Mycosis fungoides in transformation | 10/20 | (50%) |
| Anaplastic large cell lymphoma, ALK positive | 1/24 | (4%) |
| Anaplastic large cell lymphoma, ALK negative | 8/16 | (50%) |
| Peripheral T-cell lymphoma-not otherwise specified | 24/58 | (41%) |
| Angioimmunoblastic T-cell lymphoma | 12/38 | (32%) |
| **Adult T-cell leukemia-lymphoma** | **108/120** | **(90%)** |
| Others | 5/12 | (42%) |

of PTCL [13, 14] (Table 12.2). An analysis of 50 patients with PTCL-NOS revealed that CCR4-positive patients had significantly shorter survival times than those of CCR4-negative patients [14]. Furthermore, CCR4 expression increased with advancing disease stages in patients with mycosis fungoides (MF) or Sézary syndrome [15]. Although the role of CCR4 in the tumorigenesis and progression of ATL and PTCLs has not been fully elucidated, CCR4 appears to be a promising target molecule in the treatment of ATL and PTCLs.

Mogamulizumab, KW-0761, is a humanized anti-CCR4 monoclonal antibody that recognizes the N-terminal region of human CCR4 [16]. It has a defucosylated Fc region that markedly enhances antibody-dependent cell-mediated cytotoxicity (ADCC) due to increased binding affinity to the Fcγ receptor on effector cells [17]. An in vitro ADCC assay and in vivo studies in a humanized mouse model showed that mogamulizumab exhibited potent antitumor activity against ATL and PTCL cells [16, 18–20].

## *12.2.1 Clinical Efficacy of Mogamulizumab*

### 12.2.1.1 Phase I Study of Mogamulizumab for Relapsed ATL and CCR4+ PTCL in Japan

A phase I study was conducted in patients with relapsed ATL and CCR4-positive PTCL [21]. The primary objectives of this study were to assess the safety of mogamulizumab, its pharmacokinetic (PK) profile, and its maximum tolerated dose (MTD) and also determine the recommended phase II dose. The secondary objectives included the best overall response rate (ORR) and PFS. Patients received mogamulizumab by intravenous infusions once a week for 4 weeks at four dose levels (0.01, 0.1, 0.5, and 1.0 mg/kg) according to the conventional 3 + 3 design. Sixteen patients were enrolled in this phase I study, 13 of whom had ATL (11 acute type, 2 lymphoma type), 1 had MF of the tumor stage, and 2 had PTCL-not otherwise specified (PTCL-NOS). All 16 patients receiving mogamulizumab were included in the safety and efficacy analyses. No dose-limiting toxicity (DLT) was observed in any of the 13 patients who received mogamulizumab at a dose 0.01–1.0 mg/kg, and MTD was not reached. Additional three patients were enrolled to receive the highest dose of 1.0 mg/kg. The best ORR in all 16 patients was 31% (5/16; of those, 2 had complete response [CR] and 3 had partial response [PR]), and the best ORR was also 31% in patients with ATL (4/13; of those, 2 had CR and another 2 had PR). These results demonstrated the potential efficacy against relapsed ATL. Although MTD was not reached, a tendency toward increase in the incidence of grade 3 or higher toxicity was observed at 1.0 mg/kg; therefore, mogamulizumab at a dose of 1.0 mg/kg was recommended for a subsequent phase II study.

#### 12.2.1.2 Phase II Study of Mogamulizumab for Relapsed ATL in Japan

A multicenter phase II study of mogamulizumab was conducted for patients with relapsed CCR4-positive ATL [22]. The primary endpoint was ORR, and secondary endpoints included the best responses by disease sites such as peripheral blood ATL cells, skin and nodal/extranodal lesions, as well as PFS and OS. Mogamulizumab was intravenously administered once a week for 8 weeks at a dose of 1.0 mg/kg. A total of 28 patients were enrolled in this phase II study. Of these, 27 patients who received mogamulizumab were included in the safety analysis, and 26 patients, excluding 1 patient who was judged ineligible, were evaluated in the efficacy analysis. Of the 27 patients who received mogamulizumab, 14 had acute type, 6 lymphoma type, and 7 chronic type with unfavorable prognostic factors. ORR was 50% (13/26, 95% confidence interval [CI], 30–70%) including 8 CR; thus, the efficacy of mogamulizumab was confirmed. Responses according to disease sites were 100% (of 13 patients, all CR) for peripheral blood, 63% (of eight patients, three CR and two PR) for skin, and 25% (of 12 patients, 3 CR/CRu) for nodal and extranodal lesions. Median PFS and OS were 5.2 and 13.7 months, respectively. ORR was also calculated for each disease subtype, reaching 43% of patients with acute type (of 14 patients, 5 CR and 1 PR), 33% of patients with lymphoma type (of six patients, one CR and one PR), and 83% of patients with unfavorable chronic type (of six patients, two CR and three PR). Thus, these findings demonstrated that mogamulizumab induced favorable responses in patients with any disease subtype of ATL. In addition, for each age group, ORR was 39% (of 13 patients, 3 CR and 2 PR) in patients younger than 65 years and 62% (of 13 patients, 5 CR and 3 PR) in patients 65 years or older. The most common adverse events in 27 patients with ATL were lymphopenia (96%), neutropenia (52%), and thrombocytopenia (52%) as hematological toxicities and acute infusion reaction (89%), pyrexia (82%), and skin eruption (63%, 22% in grade 3/4) as non-hematological toxicities. One patient developed Stevens-Johnson syndrome (SJS), which was judged as possibly related to mogamulizumab, although that patient also received trimethoprim/sulfamethoxazole, fluconazole, and acyclovir for prevention of infection according to the protocol. These adverse events were manageable with supportive measures including corticosteroids or other drugs in all patients. These results demonstrated that mogamulizumab monotherapy showed clinically meaningful antitumor activity in patients with relapsed ATL, without an unacceptable toxicity profile.

Based on the result of this phase II study, mogamulizumab was approved for the treatment of relapsed ATL by the Japanese Pharmaceuticals and Medical Devices Agency (PMDA). However, post-marketing surveillance in Japan revealed that skin-related severe adverse events occurred in a fraction of patients with ATL. Thus, during the first 4 months after the approval by PMDA, nine skin-related severe adverse events, including four cases of SJS/toxic epidermal necrolysis (TEN), were reported, with one fatality. Therefore, a close and careful follow-up of adverse events is necessary, and the prompt use of 0.5–1.0 mg/kg prednisolone is recommended for grade 2–4 skin disorders. If SJS or TEN is suspected, methylprednisolone pulse therapy should be considered. The mechanism of skin disorders is not fully understood, but Treg reduction may contribute to skin disorders associated with the mogamulizumab treatment.

#### 12.2.1.3 Randomized Phase II Study of Mogamulizumab With or Without a Dose-Intensified Chemotherapy for Newly Diagnosed Aggressive ATL in Japan

A multicenter, randomized phase II study was conducted to examine the efficacy of the combination of mogamulizumab with a dose-intensified multidrug regimen, the so-called mLSG15, for newly diagnosed aggressive ATL [23]. In this study, patients with newly diagnosed CCR4-positive aggressive ATL were randomly assigned in a 1:1 ratio to receive mLSG15 plus mogamulizumab (arm A) or mLSG15 alone (arm B). The primary endpoint was the CR rate (%CR), and secondary endpoints included ORR, PFS, OS, and safety.

Patients received four cycles of mLSG15, with or without a total of eight cycles of mogamulizumab once every 2 weeks for 16 weeks at a dose of 1.0 mg/kg. Of the 54 randomized patients, 29 were treated in arm A and 24 in arm B. The %CR and ORR in arms A and B were 52% (15/29, 95% CI, 33–71%) vs. 33% (8/24, 95% CI, 16–55%) and 86% (25/29, 95% CI, 68–96%) vs. 75% (18/24, 95% CI, 53–90%), respectively. The %CR according to the disease site in arm A and arm B was 100% (14/14) and 43% (3/7) for peripheral blood, 92% (24/26) and 73% (16/22) for nodal and extranodal lesions, and 50% (4/8) and 60% (3/5) for skin lesions, respectively. The ORR according to the disease site in arms A and B was 100% (14/14) and 100% (7/7) for peripheral blood, 92% (24/26) and 77% (17/22) for nodal and extranodal lesions, and 75% (6/8) and 80% (4/5) for skin lesions, respectively. The median PFS in arm A and arm B was 8.5 months and 6.3 months, respectively. The median OS was not reached in both arms. The most common adverse events of any grade in each arm were neutropenia (100%, 96%), thrombocytopenia (100%, 96%), leukopenia (100%, 92%), lymphopenia (97%, 96%), anemia (97%, 92%), and febrile neutropenia (90%, 88%). Papular rush (21%), hyperglycemia (14%), pyrexia (14%), interstitial lung disease (10%), erythematous rash (7%), cytomegalovirus infection (7%), cytomegalovirus pneumonia (7%), and decreased oxygen saturation (7%) occurred only in arm A. Although mLSG15 plus mogamulizumab was found to be associated with substantial toxicities, particularly infectious and skin-related adverse events, the majority of the adverse events were manageable. These results suggested that the combination of mogamulizumab with mLSG15 may be a reasonable treatment option for managing patients with newly diagnosed aggressive ATL. However, further clinical trials are needed to confirm these results, mainly because of the small number of patients in this randomized phase II study.

## 12.3 Lenalidomide

Lenalidomide is an immunomodulatory drug (IMiD) that has been derived by altering the structure of thalidomide and was approved for multiple myeloma (MM) and myelodysplastic syndrome associated with 5q deletion in Japan. Several mechanisms of lenalidomide to boost immune response have been proposed. Lenalidomide enhances antigen uptake by antigen-presenting cells [24] and potentiates immune response by restoring dendritic cell function, inhibiting regulatory T-cell activity and activating NK cells and T cells by boosting production of interferon gamma and interleukin-2 [25]. In addition to the immunomodulatory effects, lenalidomide also has anti-angiogenic effects [26], impairs interaction between malignant cells and bone marrow stromal cells [27], induces cell cycle arrest, and has direct antiproliferative effects [28]. The antitumor activities are based on the direct interference of key pathways in tumor cells and the indirect modulation of the tumor microenvironment. In MM as well as activated B-cell type (ABC) diffuse large B-cell lymphoma (DLBCL), cereblon has been identified as the target for the immunomodulatory and antiproliferative activities of lenalidomide [29, 30]. IMiD resistance is associated with downregulation of cereblon [31], and high concentration of cereblon is associated with increased responsiveness of IMiDs [32]. In MM cells, lenalidomide-bound cereblon acquires the ability to target the proteasomal degradation of two B-cell transcription factors, IKZF1 and IKZF3, an essential step in the anti-myeloma effect [33]. In ABC-DLBCL, the tumoricidal effect of lenalidomide is associated with the cereblon-mediated downregulation of interferon regulatory factor 4 (IRF-4) leading to inhibition of the B-cell receptor signal that activates nuclear factor κappa B (NF-κB) [30]. It is considered that these mechanisms lead to clinical efficacy of lenalidomide in patients with MM and B-cell non-Hodgkin lymphoma.

On the other hand, lenalidomide has shown clinical efficacy in patients with relapsed or refractory PTCLs. The multicenter, single-arm phase II trial, the EXPECT trial, was conducted to evaluate the efficacy and safety of lenalidomide monotherapy in patients with relapsed or refractory PTCL [34]. Lenalidomide at a dose of 25 mg was orally administered once daily on days 1–21 of each 28-day cycle for a maximum of 24 months, until disease progression or development of intolerable adverse events. A total of 54 patients were enrolled in this phase II study, mostly with angioimmnoblastic T-cell lymphoma (AITL, $n = 26$, 48%) and

PTCL-NOS ($n = 20$, 37%). ORR was 22% (12/54, 95% CI, 12–36%) including CR or unconfirmed CR (CRu) in six (11%) patients. ORR was also 31% (8/26) in patients with AITL. These results demonstrated that lenalidomide monotherapy showed clinically meaningful antitumor activity in patients with heavily pretreated PTCL. However, no patients with ATL were registered in this trial.

### *12.3.1 Phase I Study of Lenalidomide for Relapsed ATL and PTCL in Japan*

A phase I study was conducted in patients with relapsed ATL and PTCL in Japan to assess the safety of lenalidomide, MTD, its PK profile, and the efficacy [35]. Dose-escalation was conducted according to the conventional 3 + 3 design. Patients in cohort 1 received oral lenalidomide 25 mg daily on days 1–21 of each 28-day cycle. Patients in cohorts 2 and 3 received 25 and 35 mg, respectively, on each day of the 28-day cycle. The treatment was continued until the development of unacceptable toxicity or disease progression.

Thirteen patients, nine of whom had ATL, and four had PTCL, were enrolled in this phase I study: three in cohort 1, six in cohort 2, and four in cohort 3. The three patients in cohort 1 received lenalidomide until disease progression without the instances of DLT. In cohort 2, one patient experienced DLT (thrombocytopenia, platelets <10,000/uL). In cohort 3, two patients had DLTs (thrombocytopenia, platelets <10,000/uL in one patient and grade 3 prolongation of QTc interval in one patient). Based on these results, 25 mg daily per 28-day cycle was regarded as the MTD in patients with ATL and PTCLs. Other grade 3 or 4 non-DLT adverse events occurring in two or more patients included neutropenia ($n = 8$), lymphopenia ($n = 7$), thrombocytopenia ($n = 3$), skin rash ($n = 3$), hyperbilirubinemia ($n = 2$), and increased aminotransaminase. Among the nine patients with ATL, three achieved PR with hematological CR in two patients, including the disappearance of skin lesions in one patient. These responses occurred between 54 and 57 days and lasted for 92, 279 + and 505 days. On the other hand, among four patients with PTCL, one achieved PR. Therefore, lenalidomide 25 mg daily on each day of the 28-day cycle was recommended for the subsequent phase II study. These results suggested the promising antitumor activity of lenalidomide in patients with ATL and PTCL. Based on the encouraging results of this phase I study, a phase II study was conducted to evaluate the efficacy of lenalidomide in patients with relapsed ATL in Japan, and patient's enrollment was completed.

## 12.4 Brentuximab Vedotin: Anti-CD30 Antibody-Drug Conjugate

CD30, a transmembrane protein from the TNF receptor family, is expressed on activated cells, and signaling via CD30 has pleiotropic effects depending on the cellular context [36]. These effects range from promotion of cell death to alteration in cell survival, activation, and differentiation. CD30 expression is highly regulated and is restricted in normal tissue to activated B and T cells; however, CD30 can also be expressed on virally infected cells. Tumor cells from various lymphocytic malignancies have also been found to express CD30. Therefore, CD30 has been considered to be an important therapeutic target for the treatment of malignant lymphomas, especially Hodgkin lymphoma and anaplastic large cell lymphoma (ALCL), because CD30 expression is higher in tumor cells of Hodgkin lymphoma and ALCL than other lymphomas. Brentuximab vedotin is an antibody-drug conjugate (ADC) containing an antimitotic drug, monomethyl auristatin E (MMAE), linked to an anti-CD30 monoclonal antibody, cAC10 [37]. Brentuximab vedotin delivers the antitubulin agent MMAE to CD30-positive malignant cells by binding specifically to CD30 on the cell surface and, after internalization, releasing MMAE inside the cell via lysosomal degradation. Because tumor cells are CD30 positive in some ATL patients, brentuximab vedotin is potentially effective for ATL.

The clinical data on brentuximab vedotin in patients with ATL is very limited. A phase I study was conducted to examine the safety and efficacy of the combination of brentuximab vedotin with multidrug regimen (cyclophosphamide, doxorubicin, prednisone (CHP)) for newly diagnosed CD30-positive PTCLs [38]. "Positive for CD30" was defined as $\geq$1% CD30 expression on malignant cells by immunohistochemistry. In this study, 39 patients were enrolled and 2 patients had ATL. The CD30-positive rate on tumor cells was 25% and 98%, respectively. These two patients with ATL received brentuximab vedotin in combination with CHP once every 3 weeks for 18 weeks at a dose of 1.8 mg/kg and achieved CR at the end of six cycles. The PFS of each patient was 7.1 and 22.8 months, respectively. Although these are results of only two patients, these results suggested the promising antitumor activity of brentuximab vedotin in patients with ATL. A randomized phase III trial is under way to compare brentuximab vedotin + CHP with CHOP (cyclophosphamide, doxorubicin, vincristine, and prednisone) for patients with newly diagnosed CD30-positive PTCLs, including CD30-positive ATL. Further investigations are warranted to evaluate the efficacy of brentuximab vedotin in patients with ATL.

## 12.5 Other Novel Agents for ATL and PTCL

Several novel agents have recently been developed for the treatment of PTCL, mainly in patients with relapsed or refractory diseases. These agents have various mechanisms of action, including a proteasome inhibitor (bortezomib), histone deacetylase inhibitors (vorinostat, romidepsin, panobinostat, belinostat, and chidamide), antifolate (pralatrexate), purine nucleoside phosphorylase inhibitor (forodesine), and biologics including antibodies and antibody-toxin conjugates (alemtuzumab, denileukin diftitox) [39]. However, the clinical data on these novel agents are mainly derived from patients with PTCL, not from ATL.

## 12.6 Conclusions

Mogamulizumab monotherapy achieved a high response rate in patients with relapsed ATL, with an acceptable toxicity profile. Available data suggest that it is one of the most active agents for ATL, and it is expected to play a key role in the treatment of ATL, especially for elderly or frail patients who are ineligible for allogeneic hematopoietic stem-cell transplantation or intensive chemotherapy. Furthermore, dose-intensified combination chemotherapy with mogamulizumab may be a reasonable treatment option for managing patients with newly diagnosed aggressive ATL. On the other hand, a reduction of the Treg subset was commonly observed in ATL patients receiving mogamulizumab and may contribute to skin disorders associated with the mogamulizumab treatment [40]. Recently, it is also considered that Treg reduction due to mogamulizumab administration may exacerbate graft-versus-host disease (GVHD) after allogeneic hematopoietic stem-cell transplantation. The mechanisms of skin adverse events and the effect of mogamulizumab on GVHD have to be analyzed more precisely. In addition, lenalidomide and brentuximab vedotin have shown the promising antitumor activity in patients with ATL. Further investigation is warranted.

## References

1. Swerdlow SH, Campo E, Harris NL, et al. WHO classification of tumors of haematopoietic and lymphoid tissues. Lyon: IARC Press; 2008.
2. Sonoda S, Li HC, Tajima K. Ethnoepidemiology of HTLV-1 related diseases: ethnic determinants of HTLV-1 susceptibility and its worldwide dispersal. Cancer Sci. 2011;102:295–301.
3. Shimoyama M. Diagnostic criteria and classification of clinical subtypes of adult T-cell leukaemia-lymphoma: a report from the Lymphoma Study Group (1984–87). Br J Haematol. 1991;79:428–37.
4. Vose J, Armitage J, Weisenburger D, International TCLP. International peripheral T-cell and natural killer/T-cell lymphoma study: pathology findings and clinical outcomes. J Clin Oncol. 2008;26:4124–30.

5. Tsukasaki K, Utsunomiya A, Fukuda H, et al. VCAP-AMP-VECP compared with biweekly CHOP for adult T-cell leukemialymphoma: Japan Clinical Oncology Group Study JCOG9801. J Clin Oncol. 2007;25:5458–64.
6. Utsunomiya A, Miyazaki Y, Takatsuka Y, et al. Improved outcome of adult T cell leukemia/ lymphoma with allogeneic hematopoietic stem cell transplantation. Bone Marrow Transplant. 2001;27:15–20.
7. Hishizawa M, Kanda J, Utsunomiya A, et al. Transplantation of allogeneic hematopoietic stem cells for adult T-cell leukemia: a nationwide retrospective study. Blood. 2010;116:1369–76.
8. Ishida T, Hishizawa M, Kato K, et al. Impact of graft-versus-host disease on allogeneic hematopoietic cell transplantation for adult T cell leukemia-lymphoma focusing on preconditioning regimens: nationwide retrospective study. Biol Blood Marrow Transplant. 2013;19:1731–9.
9. D'Ambrosio D, Iellem A, Bonecchi R, et al. Selective up-regulation of chemokine receptors CCR4 and CCR8 upon activation of polarized human type 2 Th cells. J Immunol. 1998;161:5111–5.
10. Iellem A, Mariani M, Lang R, et al. Unique chemotactic response profile and specific expression of chemokine receptors CCR4 and CCR8 by CD4(+)CD25(+) regulatory T cells. J Exp Med. 2001;194:847–53.
11. Mariani M, Lang R, Binda E, et al. Dominance of CCL22 over CCL17 in induction of chemokine receptor CCR4 desensitization and internalization on human Th2 cells. Eur J Immunol. 2004;34:231–40.
12. Ishida T, Utsunomiya A, Iida S, et al. Clinical significance of CCR4 expression in adult T-cell leukemia/lymphoma: its close association with skin involvement and unfavorable outcome. Clin Cancer Res. 2003;9:3625–34.
13. Jones D, O'Hara C, Kraus MD, et al. Expression pattern of T-cellassociated chemokine receptors and their chemokines correlates with specific subtypes of T-cell non-Hodgkin lymphoma. Blood. 2000;96:685–90.
14. Ishida T, Inagaki H, Utsunomiya A, et al. CXC chemokine receptor 3 and CC chemokine receptor 4 expression in T-cell and NK-cell lymphomas with special reference to clinicopathological significance for peripheral T-cell lymphoma, unspecified. Clin Cancer Res. 2004;10:5494–500.
15. Yagi H, Seo N, Ohshima A, et al. Chemokine receptor expression in cutaneous T cell and NK/ T-cell lymphomas: immunohistochemical staining and in vitro chemotactic assay. Am J Surg Pathol. 2006;30:1111–9.
16. Ishii T, Ishida T, Utsunomiya A, et al. Defucosylated humanized anti-CCR4 monoclonal antibody KW-0761 as a novel immunotherapeutic agent for adult T-cell leukemia/lymphoma. Clin Cancer Res. 2010;16:1520–31.
17. Shinkawa T, Nakamura K, Yamane N, et al. The absence of fucose but not the presence of galactose or bisecting N-acetylglucosamine of human IgG1 complex-type oligosaccharides shows the critical role of enhancing antibody-dependent cellular cytotoxicity. J Biol Chem. 2003;278:3466–73.
18. Yano H, Ishida T, Imada K, et al. Augmentation of antitumour activity of defucosylated chimeric anti-CCR4 monoclonal antibody in SCID mouse model of adult T-cell leukaemia/ lymphoma using G-CSF. Br J Haematol. 2008;140:586–9.
19. Niwa R, Sakurada M, Kobayashi Y, et al. Enhanced natural killer cell binding and activation by low-fucose IgG1 antibody results in potent antibody-dependent cellular cytotoxicity induction at lower antigen density. Clin Cancer Res. 2005;11:2327–36.
20. Niwa R, Shoji-Hosaka E, Sakurada M, et al. Defucosylated chimeric anti-CC chemokine receptor 4 IgG1 with enhanced antibody-dependent cellular cytotoxicity shows potent therapeutic activity to T-cell leukemia and lymphoma. Cancer Res. 2004;64:2127–33.
21. Yamamoto K, Utsunomiya A, Tobinai K, et al. Phase I study of KW-0761, a defucosylated humanized anti-CCR4 antibody, in relapsed patients with adult T-cell leukemia-lymphoma and peripheral T-cell lymphoma. J Clin Oncol. 2010;28:1591–8.

22. Ishida T, Joh T, Uike N, et al. Defucosylated anti-CCR4monoclonal antibody (KW-0761) for relapsed adult T-cell leukemia-lymphoma: a multicenter phase II study. J Clin Oncol. 2012;30:837–42.
23. Ishida T, Jo T, Takemoto S, et al. Dose-intensified chemotherapy alone or in combination with mogamulizumab in newly diagnosed aggressive adult T-cell leukaemia-lymphoma: a randomized phase II study. Br J Haematol. 2015;169:672–82.
24. Henry JY, Labarthe MC, Meyer B, et al. Enhanced cross-priming of naive CD8+ T cells by dendritic cells treated by the IMiDs(R) immunomodulatory compounds lenalidomide and pomalidomide. Immunology. 2013;139:377–85.
25. Castelli R, Cassin R, Cannavo A, et al. Immunomodulatory drugs: new options for the treatment of myelodysplastic syndromes. Clin Lymphoma Myeloma Leuk. 2013;13:1–7.
26. Martiniani R, Di Loreto V, Di Sano C, et al. Biological activity of lenalidomide and its underlying therapeutic effects in multiple myeloma. Adv Hematol. 2012;2012:842945.
27. Mitsiades CS, Mitsiades NS, Richardson PG, et al. Multiple myeloma: a prototypic disease model for the characterization and therapeutic targeting of interactions between tumor cells and their local microenvironment. J Cell Biochem. 2007;101:950–68.
28. Verhelle D, Corral LG, Wong K, et al. Lenalidomide and CC-4047 inhibit the proliferation of malignant B cells while expanding normal CD34+ progenitor cells. Cancer Res. 2007;67:746–55.
29. Lopez-Girona A, Mendy D, Ito T, et al. Cereblon is a direct protein target for immunomodulatory and antiproliferative activities of lenalidomide and pomalidomide. Leukemia. 2012;26:2326–35.
30. Zhang LH, Kosek J, Wang M, et al. Lenalidomide efficacy in activated B-cell-like subtype diffuse large B-cell lymphoma is dependent upon IRF4 and cereblon expression. Br J Haematol. 2013;160:487–502.
31. Zhu YX, Braggio E, Shi CX, et al. Cereblon expression is required for the antimyeloma activity of lenalidomide and pomalidomide. Blood. 2011;118:4771–9.
32. Heintel D, Rocci A, Ludwig H, et al. High expression of cereblon (CRBN) is associated with improved clinical response in patients with multiple myeloma treated with lenalidomide and dexamethasone. Br J Haematol. 2013;161:695–700.
33. Lu G, Middleton RE, Sun H, et al. The myeloma drug lenalidomide promotes the cereblon-dependent destruction of Ikaros proteins. Science. 2014;343:305–9.
34. Morschhauser F, Fitoussi O, Haioun C, et al. A phase 2, multicentre, single-arm, open-label study to evaluate the safety and efficacy of single-agent lenalidomide (Revlimid) in subjects with relapsed or refractory peripheral T-cell non-Hodgkin lymphoma: the EXPECT trial. Eur J Cancer. 2013;49:2869–76.
35. Uike N, Ogura M, Imaizumi Y, et al. Multicenter phase I dose-escalation study of lenalidomide in patients with relapsed adult T-cell leukemia-lymphoma (ATL) or peripheral T-cell lymphoma (PTCL). [abstract 2737]. Presented at the 54th Annual Meeting of the American Society of Hematology. Atlanta, USA; December 8–11, 2012.
36. Deutsch YE, Tadmor T, Podack ER, Rosenblatt JD. CD30: an important new target in hematologic malignancies. Leuk Lymphoma. 2011;52:1641–54.
37. Vaklavas C, Forero-Torres A. Safety and efficacy of brentuximab vedotin in patients with Hodgkin lymphoma or systemic anaplastic large cell lymphoma. Ther Adv Hematol. 2012;3:209–25.
38. Fanale MA, Horwitz SM, Forero-Torres A, et al. Brentuximab vedotin in the front-line treatment of patients with CD30+ peripheral T-cell lymphomas: results of a phase I study. J Clin Oncol. 2014;32:3137–43.
39. Foss FM, Zinzani PL, Vose JM, Gascoyne RD, Rosen ST, Tobinai K. Peripheral T-cell lymphoma. Blood. 2011;117:6756–67.
40. Ishida T, Ito A, Sato F, et al. Stevens-Johnson syndrome associated with mogamulizumab treatment of adult T-cell leukemia/lymphoma. Cancer Sci. 2013;104:647–50.

# Chapter 13
# Prevention of Human T-Cell Leukemia Virus Type 1 (HTLV-1) Mother-to-Child Transmission

**Kiyonori Miura and Hideaki Masuzaki**

## 13.1 Human T-Cell Leukemia Virus Type 1 (HTLV-1)-Related Diseases

Worldwide, there are an estimated 20 million people infected with human T-cell leukemia virus type 1 (HTLV-1) [1]. The main regions with endemic HTLV-1 are the southern part of Japan, sub-Saharan Africa, South America, the Caribbean region, and specific regions in the Middle East and Australo-Melanesian populations [2].

HTLV-1 causes adult T-cell leukemia-lymphoma (ATL) and HTLV-1-associated myelopathy (HAM) in a small proportion of HTLV-1 carriers, after a long incubation period. Improving knowledge on the epidemiology of HTLV-1-associated diseases demonstrates why HTLV-1 prevention is necessary.

### *13.1.1 Adult T-Cell Leukemia-Lymphoma*

Adult T-cell leukemia-lymphoma (ATL) is a malignancy of peripheral T-cell lymphocytes, caused by HTLV-1 infection. The number of HTLV-1 carriers who develop ATL is estimated at 1200 annually, and the lifetime risk for ATL in HTLV-1 carriers is approximately 5% [3]. The median survival time of people with ATL is under 12 months [5], and currently there is no vaccine available. When acute transformation of ATL occurs, chemotherapy is the first choice of medical treatment. To date, various chemotherapy protocols have been used to treat aggressive

K. Miura (✉) • H. Masuzaki
Departments of Obstetrics and Gynecology, Nagasaki University Graduate School of Biomedical Sciences, 1-7-1 Sakamoto, Nagasaki 852-8501, Japan
e-mail: kiyonori@nagasaki-u.ac.jp

 
T. Watanabe, T. Fukushima (eds.), *Adult T-cell Leukemia/Lymphoma*,
DOI 10.1007/978-4-431-56523-9_13

ATL in Japan [4]; however, ATL is difficult to cure and presently has a poor prognosis. The median age of onset is 67 years, indicating a long latent period from initial infection with HTLV-1 to the onset of ATL. The majority of ATL cases develop from cases of HTLV-1 infection acquired in childhood, through vertical transmission from mother to child, rather than in adult life (through blood transfusions or sexual transmission) [6, 7].

### *13.1.2 HTLV-1-Associated Myelopathy*

HTLV-1-associated myelopathy (HAM), which can develop after an incubation period of several years (mean age at onset is 40–50 years), is characterized by serious neurological clinical signs, including spasticity and/or hyperreflexia of the lower extremities, urinary bladder disturbance, lower extremity muscle weakness, and sensory disturbances with lower back pain. The lifetime risk of HAM in HTLV-1 carriers is 0.25% in Japan [6, 7] and 1.9% in Jamaica and Trinidad [8]. In a prospective study in the United States (USA), 3.7% of HTLV-1 carriers were diagnosed with HAM [9]. Major symptoms for individuals with HTLV-1 include pain, sensory-motor dysfunction, and urinary symptoms. To date, various therapies have been used to try and improve patients' quality of life; however, there is no cure for this disease.

It is important to recognize that there are no effective vaccines against HTLV-1 and no medication or therapies that will cure HTLV-1-related diseases. Therefore, primary prevention of mother-to-child transmission of HTLV-1 infection is the only effective strategy likely to reduce HTLV-1 carrier status and HTLV-1-related diseases in the next generation.

## 13.2 Infection Routes of HTLV-1

HTLV-1 has three modes of transmission: (1) vertically, from mother to child, antenatal or postnatal, predominantly linked with prolonged breastfeeding; (2) sexual intercourse, mainly occurring from male to female; and (3) blood-borne transmission. In addition, transmission through intravenous drug use is also possible [7]. Routine HTLV-1 screening of blood donations has been performed in Japan and many other countries, to prevent blood transfusion-related HTLV-1 transmission. Since 2011, HTLV-1 screening of pregnant women has been recommended in Japan [10].

## 13.3 Mother-to-Child Transmission Through Breastfeeding

HTLV-1 is primarily transmitted vertically from mother to child. In Nagasaki, an HTLV-1-endemic area in Northern Kyushu, Japan, several studies supporting the possibility of breast milk-borne transmission include (1) HTLV-1 antigens identified in breast milk from HTLV-1 carriers; (2) oral administration of fresh human breast milk from HTLV-1 carriers to uninfected marmosets causing transmission; (3) retrospective data showing an increased rate of HTLV-1 infection in breast milk-fed children, compared with bottle milk-fed children; and (4) prospective data showing that prevalence of mother-to-child transmission was 20.5% in a group of mothers that breastfed for 6 months or longer, 8.3% in a group that breastfed for less than 6 months, and 2.4% in a group that bottle-fed (Fig. 13.1). The above studies have provided important information; breastfeeding is associated with mother-to-child transmission of HTLV-1, but breast milk-borne transmission is not the only route of transmission. A longer duration of breastfeeding increases the risk of mother-to-child transmission, whereas bottle-feeding could reduce this risk [7, 11]. To reduce the prevalence of HTLV-1 carriers and prevent further development of HTLV-1-related diseases in the next generation, routine HTLV-1 screening of pregnant women is essential [7, 11].

Several studies in other regions and countries support these Nagasaki studies. In Kagoshima (an endemic area in southern Kyushu, Japan), an epidemiological study identified the prevalence of mother-to-child transmission to be 25.0% in a group that breastfed for 7 months or longer (long-term breastfeeding), 3.8% in a group

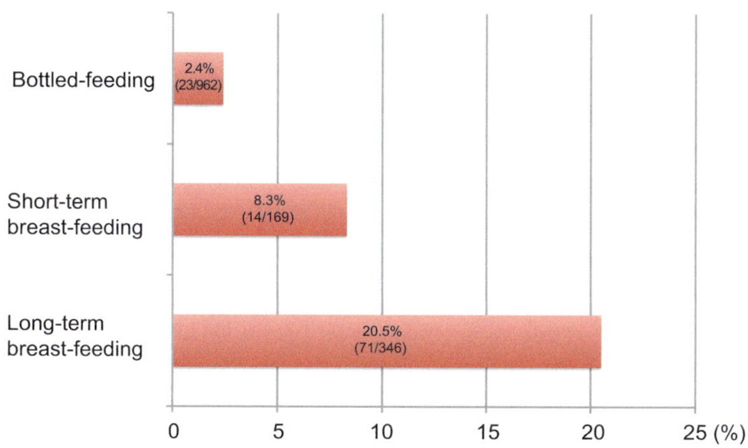


**Fig. 13.1** Prevalence of mother-to-child transmission of HTLV-1 for each feeding method. The prevalence of mother-to-child transmission was 20.5% in the group of long-term breastfeeding, 8.3% in the group of the short-term breastfeeding, and 2.4% in the group of bottle-feeding. Long-term breastfeeding is defined as a duration of 6 months or longer, while short-term breastfeeding is defined as a duration of less than 6 months

that breastfed for less than 7 months (short-term breastfeeding), and 5.6% in a group that bottle-fed [12]. There was a significant difference between the short-term and long-term breastfeeding groups. In Jamaica, in children observed for at least 24 months, the prevalence of mother-to-child transmission was 32% in the group that was breastfed for 12 months or longer and 9% in the group that was breastfed for less than 12 months [13]. Compared with children who were breastfed for 12 months or less, relative risk in children who were breastfed for 12 to 18 months was 6.4 and for those who were breastfed for longer than 18 months was 18.1 [13].

As previously noted, with the vertical transmission of HTLV-1 from mother to child, a longer duration of breastfeeding increases the risk of transmission [7, 11]. The most effective time to prevent vertical transmission of HTLV-1 is at birth. To provide a choice of feeding methods for babies born to HTLV-1 carriers, antenatal screening for HTLV-1 has been carried out in Nagasaki since 1987 [7, 11] and has also been proposed in Europe and Jamaica. In Japan, the estimated number of HTLV-1 carriers in 2007 was 1.08 million [14, 15]. The number of HTLV-1 carriers in each region has been estimated to be 492,582 in Kyushu, 171,843 in Kinki, and 190,609 in Kanto. Between 1990 and 2007, the prevalence of HTLV-1 carriers in Kyushu decreased significantly from 50.9% in 1990 to 45.7% in 2007, while those in the metropolitan areas (Kinki and Kanto regions) increased from 10.8% in 1990 to 17.7% in 2007 [14, 15]. These changes were considered to be mainly because of migration from Kyushu to the metropolitan areas [14, 15]. HTLV-1 carriers are distributed across the whole country, and primary prevention is the only effective strategy to reduce HTLV-1 carriers in the next generation; therefore, to prevent mother-to-child transmission of HTLV-1, nationwide antenatal screening for HTLV-1 has been implemented since 2011 in Japan [10].

## 13.4 Prevention of Vertical Transmission of HTLV-1 at Birth

### *13.4.1 Bottle-Feeding*

It is important to emphasize that HTLV-1-associated diseases are only caused by HTLV-1 carriers, and people who are seronegative for HTLV-1 will never develop HTLV-1-associated diseases. Furthermore, it is not possible to prevent the development of ATL or other HTLV-1-associated disorders in carriers. To date, no HTLV-1 vaccine has reached clinical trial stage. The majority of HTLV-1 infections are through mother-to-child transmission, and in general, ATL only develops from HTLV-1 carriers infected in childhood [7, 11]. Bottle-feeding has demonstrated a reduction in the prevalence of mother-to-child transmission from 20.5% to 2.4% [7, 11]. In Japan, primary prevention of mother-to-child transmission of HTLV-1 infection is the only effective strategy likely to reduce HTLV-1 carrier status and HTLV-1-related diseases in the next generation, despite the loss of health benefits associated with breastfeeding. Because breastfeeding can improve infant mortality rates in some developing countries, this prevention strategy for HTLV-1 may be controversial, and implementation will be dependent on pregnancy status and/or medical situations in each country [7].

### 13.4.2 Two Alternative Feeding Methods to Reduce the Risk of Breastmilk HTLV-1 Transmission

In Nagasaki, bottle-feeding is recommended as the best feeding method to prevent mother-to-child transmission of HTLV-1 [7, 11]. Conversely, in Kagoshima, HTLV-1-positive mothers are advised to bottle-feed or breastfeed short term [16]. In general, most pregnant women seem to believe that breastfeeding has positive effects for the health of both baby and mother. Therefore, HTLV-1-carrier mothers want to choose breastfeeding for their babies. There are two alternative breastfeeding methods to reduce the risk of HTLV-1 vertical transmission, one is freeze-thawing breast milk, and the other is short-term breastfeeding.

Freeze-thawing breast milk disrupts HTLV-1-infected cells in vitro and seems to reduce the rate of mother-to-child transmission. However, freeze-thawing breast milk is a difficult feeding method for many mothers, as breast milk should be frozen at −20 °C or below for 12 h or longer. Conversely, several studies, as noted above, demonstrated that short-term breastfeeding could also reduce the rate of mother-to-child transmission of HTLV-1. In particular, a study in Kagoshima suggested that short-term breastfeeding (<3 months) and bottle-feeding showed almost the same protective effect in reducing mother-to-child transmission of HTLV-1 [16].

Based on the benefit of breastfeeding and the risk of mother-to-child transmission of HTLV-1 in alternative feeding methods, some HTLV-1-positive pregnant women choose short-term breastfeeding or freeze-thawing breast milk in Japan. In addition, other reasons also may affect their decision to select alternative breastfeeding methods including: (1) medical staff (gynecologists, pediatricians, midwives, and public health nurses) might strongly recommend breastfeeding, based on its benefits, (2) HTLV-1-positive mothers might be concerned that their family and/or neighbors will become aware of their carrier status if they decide not to breastfeed, and (3) some mothers might continue to breastfeed because of their economic situation.

## 13.5 Current Strategy in Japan to Prevent Mother-to-Child Transmission of HTLV-1

Since 2011, it is recommended that all pregnant women in Japan are screened for HTLV-1 by particle agglutination (PA) or chemiluminescent enzyme immunoassay (CLEIA) [7, 10, 11].

In Nagasaki, the committee for the ATL Prevention Program Nagasaki has been established since 1987 [17]. The establishment of a committee is recommended to promote HTLV-1 prevention programs. The latest version of the prevention protocol for HTLV-1 mother-to-child transmission in Nagasaki is shown in Fig. 13.2 [7]. It is important to highlight that both PA and CLEIA have high sensitivity and specificity, but there is still the possibility of false-positive results, especially in non-endemic areas [18]. When PA or CLEIA tests show positive or pseudo-positive results, Western blotting should also be performed to confirm results. However, Western blots can also show indeterminate results. Therefore, for a definitive result, polymerase chain reaction (PCR) analysis to detect HTLV-1 provirus DNA is performed as an additional confirmation test. In Nagasaki, as the best system to screen HTLV-1 carriers, Western blots in combination with PCR tests seem to be more useful than Western blot tests alone. In Nagasaki, since 2011, for pregnant women with inconclusive results by Western blot, a PCR has been performed as an additional confirmation test. PCR

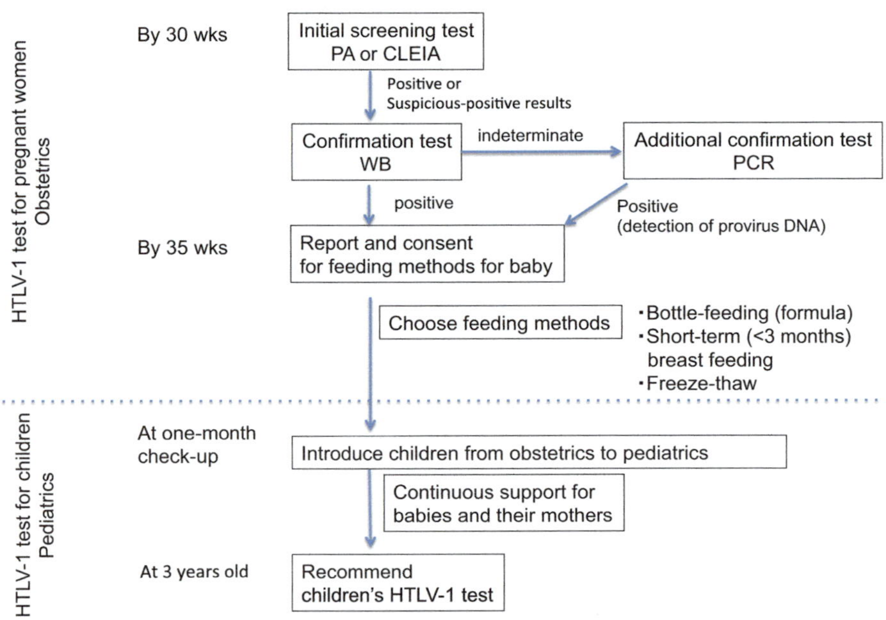


**Fig. 13.2** Prevention protocol for HTLV-1 mother-to-child transmission in Nagasaki, Japan. In Nagasaki, the committee of adult T-cell leukemia-lymphoma (ATL) Prevention Program Nagasaki has been established since 1987. This is the latest version of prevention protocol in Nagasaki. *CLEIA* chemiluminescence enzyme immunoassay, *PA* particle agglutination, *WB* Western blot

primers and probes for real-time PCR have been designed for the pX region of HTLV-1, because this region is conserved between HTLV-1 subtypes.

When advising on HTLV-1 infection during pregnancy, pregnant women with HTLV-1 infections receive detailed information about HTLV-1, mother-to-child transmission, and clinical significance, to prevent the vertical transmission of HTLV-1. Except for HTLV-1-positive women with high-risk babies, e.g., premature or severe fetal growth restrictions, all pregnant women with HTLV-1 infection are advised to undertake exclusive bottle-feeding, freeze-thawing of breast milk, or short-term breastfeeding (<3 months). Continuous support for HTLV-1-carrier mothers is critical, especially for those who have chosen the latter two feeding options. In Nagasaki, at 1-month checkups, obstetricians introduce the babies born from HTLV-1-carrier mothers to pediatricians, to support HTLV-1-positive mothers and their babies. For the children born from HTLV-1-positive mothers, it is recommended that an HTLV-1 test is performed at 3 years old.

## 13.6 Importance of Educating Medical Staff in the Prevention of Vertical Transmission of HTLV-1

Education of medical staff (obstetricians, pediatricians, midwives, and public health nurses) is essential [11]. If medical staff do not understand the severity of HTLV-1-related diseases, it is difficult to deliver the appropriate information to pregnant women and to explain the significance of preventing HTLV-1 transmission [11].

In Nagasaki, to prevent mother-to-child transmission, HTLV-1 carriers are advised to undertake bottle-feeding as a first choice and short-term breastfeeding (for a maximum of 3 months) or freeze-thawing breast milk as second choice.

Medical staff in Nagasaki recognize that bottle-feeding is the most reliable and effective method to reduce the risk of breast milk-borne transmission of HTLV-1. However, the prevalence of HTLV-1 carriers selecting bottle-feeding decreased from 79.1% in 1999 to 59.4% in 2008. If medical staff have no experience of encountering ATL, they may think it is treatable like other leukemias (e.g., acute lymphoblastic leukemia, acute lymphocytic leukemia, malignant lymphoma), and the incidence of ATL in carriers would be low. In our experience, most pregnant women visiting doctors select breastfeeding rather than bottle-feeding, probably because they believe breastfeeding is the most important tool for rearing babies. Conversely, HTLV-1-carrier mothers may be concerned about confidentiality. Education of medical staff and the community is important, so consequently, to raise awareness in medical staff that ATL is still difficult to cure, and prevention of mother-to-child transmission of HTLV-1 is important, we implemented annual workshops as part of the ATL prevention program. In these workshops, medical staff working on the prevention program listened to the experiences of patients with HTLV-1-related diseases, the current state of ATL/HAM treatment in hematology and current HTLV-1 research. An increase in awareness in medical staff was reflected in an increase in the rate of the bottle-feeding selected by HTLV-1 carriers, with a prevalence of 75.8% in 2013 (manuscript in preparation). For the prevention of HTLV-1 mother-to-child transmission, education about HTLV-1 and related diseases can heighten the awareness of medical staff [11].

## 13.7 Importance of Follow-Up for HTLV-1-Carrier Mothers and Their Babies

As mentioned previously, in the HTLV-1 mother-to-child transmission prevention program, there were serious problems economically, emotionally, and socially. Recently, the difficulty of weaning from the breast has been recognized as a serious problem with short-term breastfeeding [7, 16]. In Kagoshima, approximately 12.5% of mothers who had chosen short-term breastfeeding failed to wean their babies as scheduled [16]. Therefore, supporting HTLV-1-positive mothers to stop breastfeeding within the 3-month period is important. In Kagoshima, visits by public health nurses are standard and they determine if mothers need the support of midwives [16].

## 13.8 Agenda for the Future

PCR tests for HTLV-1 provirus DNA were performed in umbilical cord-blood samples of babies born to carrier mothers. None of the babies who were positive in the cord blood were still positive in peripheral blood at 6 months after birth [19]. Conversely, all babies who were diagnosed as HTLV-1 carriers beyond 12 months of age had been PCR negative in their cord blood [19]. Therefore, intrauterine transmission of HTLV-1 may be rare.

When HTLV-1-positive mothers chose to bottle-feed, mother-to-child transmission of HTLV-1 was identified in 2.4% of babies, suggesting other routes of vertical transmission antenatally or postnatally [7, 11]. In addition, previous studies reported that vertical transmission of HTLV-1 was associated with higher maternal HTLV-1 antibody titer or provirus load in blood or breast milk, prolonged duration of ruptured membranes during delivery, and lower maternal income [13, 20, 21].

In the future, to develop the best prevention protocol for HTLV-1 mother-to-child transmission, the following needs to be clarified: (1) the secondary pathway of HTLV-1 mother-to-child transmission, e.g., transmission during delivery and transplacental transmission, (2) association between clinical findings during pregnancy and the risk of mother-to-child transmission, (3) association between HTLV-1 provirus load in carrier mothers and the risk of mother-to-child transmission, (4) association between HTLV-1 provirus load in carrier mothers and the future development of ATL, and (5) the possibility of a vaccine for HTLV-1 in endemic areas. In addition to the prevention of HTLV-1 mother-to-child transmission, for the obstetric care for pregnant women with HTLV-1 infection, effectiveness of avoiding fetal invasive monitoring and iatrogenic rupture of membranes, the influence of maternal proviral load, and the mode of delivery should be also clarified [22].

## 13.9 Lessons from the Cases in the Nagasaki HTLV-1 Prevention Program

We have experienced several difficult cases in the prevention program; critical points learned from these cases are summarized here.

**Case 1: The Aim of HTLV-1 Screening in Pregnant Women**
A pregnant woman (gravida 0, para 0) was diagnosed as an HTLV-1 carrier during the standard screening for HTLV-1 infection in pregnant women. After counseling regarding feeding methods, the husband and pregnant woman's mother were also tested to identify the route of transmission; however, the tests were negative. Consequently, the pregnant woman and her husband separated. Before the HTLV-1 screening test is performed, we explain to parents that HTLV-1 screening in pregnant women is for their baby's health, because the aim of this prevention protocol is to reduce HTLV-1 carriers and HTLV-1-related diseases in the next generation. In the HTLV-1 screening of pregnant women, we do not recommend testing grandmothers, because there is the possibility for additional concerns within the family. Furthermore, it was revealed during the medical interview there was the possibility that this pregnant woman received donated milk at birth. Therefore, the community of obstetricians, midwives, and neonatologists should pay attention to the issue of donated milk, and donated milk should be also screened for HTLV-1 infection [23].

**Case 2: Sexual Transmission from Husband to Wife**
A pregnant woman (gravida 1, para 1) was diagnosed as HTLV-1 negative during her first pregnancy. However, in her second pregnancy, the PA test identified a positive result. Therefore, a Western blot test was performed as a confirmation test, which was indeterminate. Consequently, a PCR was performed, and a very low proviral load of HTLV-1 was detected. The pregnant woman's mother was HTLV-1 negative, but her husband was positive, suggesting sexual transmission from husband to wife. Other studies have reported that more than half of cases (6/11) of husband-to-wife transmission were between 1 and 4 years after marriage [24]. Therefore, we recommend that the HTLV-1 screening test should be performed for each pregnancy. In future studies, to gather more detailed data regarding HTLV-1 carriers with a low HTLV-1 provirus load, we have to clarify

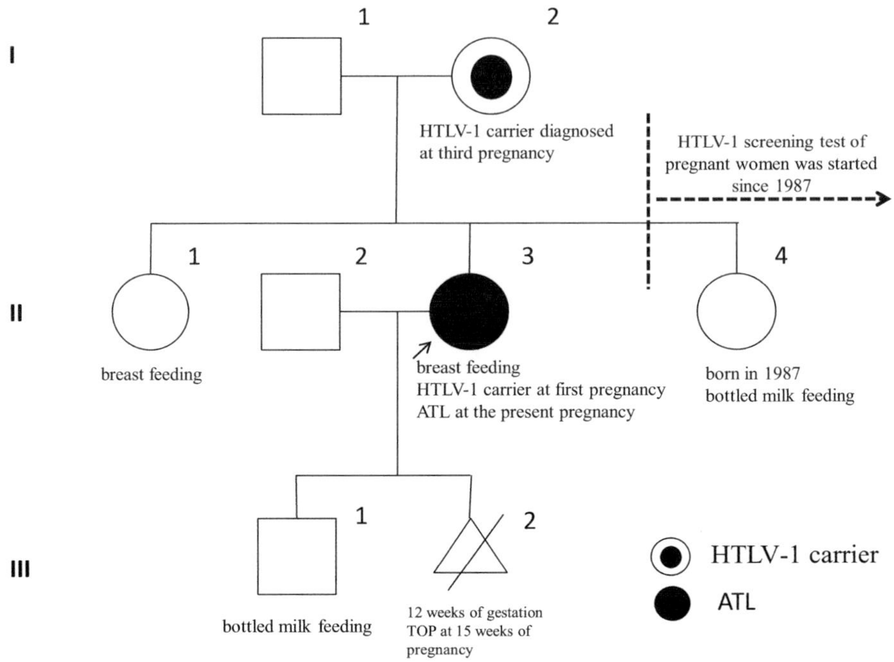


**Fig. 13.3** Family tree of pregnant woman with adult T-cell leukemia-lymphoma. The present case (II-3) was breastfed and became an HTLV-1 carrier via mother-to-child transmission. When her younger sister (II-4) was born in 1987, her mother (I-2) was diagnosed with HTLV-1. To reduce the risk of mother-to-child transmission of HTLV-1, her younger sister (II-4) was bottle-fed, and she did not become an HTLV-1 carrier. During her first pregnancy, the present case (II-3) was diagnosed as an HTLV-1 carrier by screening, and she chose to bottle-feed her first child (III-1). Her first child was confirmed as HTLV-1 negative. When her first child was 8 years old, the present case (II-3) was diagnosed with unfavorable chronic ATL at 12 weeks' gestation (Reused from Ref. [24] with permission)

if a very low HTLV-1 provirus load can cause mother-to-child transmission of HTLV-1 and lead on to the development of HTLV-1-related diseases.

**Case 3: ATL in a Pregnant Woman Diagnosed as an HTLV-1 Carrier**

We have experienced ATL in a pregnant woman with HTLV-1 [25]. A family tree of the present case (II-3), who was diagnosed with ATL during pregnancy, is shown in Fig. 13.3. In Nagasaki, screening for HTLV-1 in all pregnant women has been implemented since 1987 [7, 11]. As a result, for the first time, a grandmother (I-2) had a diagnosis of being an HTLV-1 carrier at her fourth pregnancy (II-4) in 1987. Therefore, her younger sister (II-4) received bottled milk to avoid mother-to-child transmission of HTLV-1. The present case (II-3), who was born before 1987, became an HTLV-1 carrier because alternative feeding methods were not recommended. When the present case (II-3) was pregnant with her first child (III-1), HTLV-1 infection was detected by screening, and she selected bottle-

**Table 13.1** Five cases of adult T-cell leukemia–lymphoma (ATL) during pregnancy (Modified from Ref. [24] with permission)

| Case no. | Country | Age (years) | Gestational weeks at diagnosis of ATL | Clinical variant of ATL | Clinical course after diagnosis of ATL |
|---|---|---|---|---|---|
| 1[28] | Japan | 28 | 38 | Acute | At 6 months after delivery, she died despite chemotherapy |
| 2[29] | Japan | 43 | 30 | Acute | At 4 weeks after delivery, she died despite chemotherapy |
| 3[30] | USA | 23 | 26 | Acute | At 3 days after delivery, she died because of widespread disease |
| 4[31] | USA | 27 | 28 | Acute | Chemotherapy was performed and she was discharged after a 4-week hospital stay. Subsequently, hemato-poietic stem cell transplantation was considered |
| 5 (Case 3)[26] | Japan | 30 | 12 | Unfavorable chronic | Within 1 year after TOP, she died despite medical treatment |

*TOP* termination of pregnancy

feeding. When her child was 3 years old, he (III-1) was confirmed as HTLV-1 negative. This family history highlights the significance of HTLV-1 screening in pregnant women.

During the second pregnancy of the present case, she had a persistent fever and cough at 8 weeks' gestation. From the detailed hematological examination, she was diagnosed with chronic ATL with unfavorable prognostic factors for survival, defined by one or more of the following clinical factors: low serum albumin, high lactate dehydrogenase (LDH), or high blood urea nitrogen (BUN) levels [26, 27]. The median survival time for chronic ATL cases with unfavorable prognostic factors is about 15 months [27]. Once ATL progresses to acute crisis, the median survival time is approximately 1 year [28]. To date, five cases of ATL during pregnancy have been reported (Table 13.1), all of which had a poor prognosis despite medical treatment [25, 29–32].

## 13.10 Conclusion

There are an estimated 1.08 million HTLV-1 carriers in Japan [14]. ATL and other HTLV-1-related diseases are still difficult to cure and currently have a poor prognosis. Therefore, to reduce ATL and HTLV-1-related diseases in the next generation, especially in endemic areas, HTLV-1 screening in pregnant women is an important step in preventing mother-to-child transmission of HTLV-1 infection [7, 11].

## References

1. De Thé G, Kazanji M. J Acquir Immune Defic Syndr Hum Retrovirol. 1996;13(Suppl 1): S191–8.
2. Gessain A, Cassar O. Epidemiological aspects and world distribution of HTLV-1 infection. Front Microbiol. 2012;15(3):388.
3. Tajima K. The 4th nationwide study of adult T-cell leukemia/lymphoma (ATL) in Japan: estimates of risk of ATL and its geographical and clinical features. The T- and B-cell Malignancy Study Group. Int J Cancer. 1990;45:237–43.
4. Katsuya H, Yamanaka T, Ishitsuka K, et al. Prognostic index for acute- and lymphoma-type adult T-cell leukemia/lymphoma. J Clin Oncol. 2012;30(14):1635–40.
5. Tsukasaki K, Tobinai K. Biology and treatment of HTLV-1 associated T-cell lymphomas. Best Pract Res Clin Haematol. 2013;26:3–14.
6. Yamaguchi K, Watanabe T, Uchimaru K et al. A guidance for HTLV-1 carriers. Ministry of Health, Labour and Welfare, Tokyo. Available via: http://www.mhlw.go.jp/bunya/kenkou/kekkaku-kansenshou19/dl/htlv-1_d.pdf. Accessed 22 Apr 2016 (in Japanese).
7. Moriuchi H, Masuzaki H, Doi H, et al. Mother-to-child transmission of human T-cell lymphotropic virus type 1. Pediatr Infect Dis J. 2013;32(2):175–7.
8. De Thé G, Bomford R. An HTLV-1 vaccine: why, how, for whom? AIDS Res Hum Retrovir. 1993;9:381–6.
9. Hino S, Katamine MH, et al. Primary prevention of HTLV-1 in Japan. Leukemia. 1997;11 (Suppl 3):57–9.
10. Minakami H, Maeda T, Fujii T. Guidelines for obstetrical practice in Japan: Japan Society of Obstetrics and Gynecology (JSOG) and Japan Association of Obstetricians and Gynecologists (JAOG) 2014 edition. J Obstet Gynaecol Res. 2014;40:1469–99.
11. Hino S. Establishment of the milk-borne transmission as a key factor for the peculiar endemicity of human T-lymphotropic virus type 1 (HTLV-1): the ATL Prevention Program Nagasaki. Proc Jpn Acad Ser B Phys Biol Sci. 2011;87:152–66.
12. Oki T, Yoshinaga M, Otsuka H. Asero-epidemiological study on mother-to-child transmission of HTLV-I in southern Kyushu, Japan. Asia Ocean J Obstet Gynaecol. 1992;18(4):371–7.
13. Wiktor SZ, Pate EJ, Rosenberg PS, et al. Mother-to-child transmission of human T-cell lymphotropic virus type I associated with prolonged breast-feeding. J Hum Virol. 1997;1 (1):37–44.
14. Satake M, Yamaguchi K, Tadokoro K. Current prevalence of HTLV-1 in Japan as determined by screening of blood donors. J Med Virol. 2012;84:327–35.
15. Watanabe T. Current status of HTLV-1 infection. Int J Hematol. 2011;94:430–4.
16. Nerome Y, Kojyo K, Ninomiya Y, et al. Current human T-cell lymphotropic virus type 1 mother-to-child transmission prevention status in Kagoshima. Pediatr Int. 2014;56(4):640–3.
17. The Committee of ATL Prevention Program Nagasaki (APP Nagasaki), Child Welfare Bureau of Nagasaki Prefecture. Report of joint study on the prevention of ATL by blocking mother-to-child transmission of HTLV-1: experiences and perspectives of 20 years. Nagasaki: Nagasaki Prefecture; 2008. p. 1–21. (in Japanese)
18. Hanaoka M, Kubo T, Saitoh A. Discrepancy between human T-cell lymphotropic virus type I screening test and confirmatory tests in non-endemic areas. J Obstet Gynaecol Res. 2012;38:793–6.
19. Katamine S, Moriuchi R, Yamamoto T, et al. HTLV-I proviral DNA in umbilical cord blood of babies born to carrier mothers. Lancet. 1994;343(8909):1326–7.
20. Ureta-Vidal A, Angelin-Duclos C, Tortevoye P, et al. Mother-to-child transmission of human T-cell-leukemia/lymphoma virus type I: implication of high antiviral antibody titer and high proviral load in carrier mothers. Int J Cancer. 1999;82(6):832–6.
21. Li HC, Biggar RJ, Miley WJ, et al. Provirus load in breast milk and risk of mother-to-child transmission of human T lymphotropic virus type I. J Infect Dis. 2004;190(7):1275–8.

22. Carneiro-Proietti AB, Amaranto-Damasio MS, Leal-Horiguchi CF, et al. Mother-to-child transmission of human T-Cell lymphotropic viruses-1/2: what we know, and what are the gaps in understanding and preventing this route of infection. J Pediatr Infect Dis Soc. 2014;3 (Suppl 1):S24–9.
23. Rigourd V, Meyer V, Kieffer F, et al. HTLV and "donating" milk. Bull Soc Pathol Exot. 2011;104(3):205–8.
24. Take H, Umemoto M, Kusuhara K, et al. Transmission routes of HTLV-I: an analysis of 66 families. Jpn J Cancer Res. 1993;84(12):1265–7.
25. Fuchi N, Miura K, Imaizumi Y, et al. Adult T-cell leukemia-lymphoma in a pregnant woman diagnosed as a human T-cell lymphotropic virus type 1 carrier. J Obstet Gynaecol Res. 2016;42(3):336–40.
26. Shimoyama M. Diagnostic criteria and classification of clinical subtypes of adult T-cell leukaemia-lymphoma. A report from the Lymphoma Study Group (1984–87). Br J Haematol. 1991;79:428–37.
27. Shimoyama M. Chemotherapy of ATL. In: Takatsuki K, editor. Adult T-cell leukemia. Oxford: Oxford University Press; 1994. p. 221–37.
28. Takasaki Y, Iwanaga M, Imaizumi Y, et al. Long-term study of indolent adult T-cell leukemia–lymphoma. Blood. 2010;115:4337–43.
29. Ohba T, Matsuo I, Katabuchi H, et al. Adult T-cell leukemia/lymphoma in pregnancy. Obstet Gynecol. 1988;72:445–7.
30. Utsumi T, Tsuda A, Hirano H, et al. A case of pregnancy with adult T-cell leukemia. J Obstet Gynaecol Res. 1996;22:599–601.
31. Safdar A, Johnson N, Gonzalez F, et al. Adult T-cell leukemia–lymphoma during pregnancy. N Engl J Med. 2002;346:2014–5.
32. Amor MM, Olaso AS, Atienza R, et al. Adult T-cell leukemia–lymphoma during pregnancy. Case Rep Oncol Med doi. 2013; doi:10.1155/2013/631825.

MIX
Papier aus verantwortungsvollen Quellen
Paper from responsible sources
FSC® C105338

If you have any concerns about our products,
you can contact us on
**ProductSafety@springernature.com**

In case Publisher is established outside the EU,
the EU authorized representative is:
**Springer Nature Customer Service Center GmbH**
**Europaplatz 3, 69115 Heidelberg, Germany**

Printed by Libri Plureos GmbH
in Hamburg, Germany